HEALING FOOD

— FOR —

COMMON AILMENTS

Dr Penny Stanway

A GAIA ORIGINAL

Gaia Books Limited

A GAIA ORIGINAL

Written by Dr Penny Stanway

Based on an idea by Joss Pearson

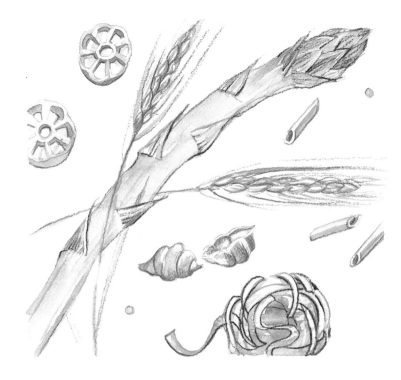

Photography	Peter Warren
Editorial	Joanna Godfrey Wood
Design	Helen Spencer
	Sara Mathews
Illustration	Debbie Hinks
Production	Susan Walby

GAIA

® This is a Registered Trade Mark
of Gaia Books Limited
This edition first published in the United Kingdom
in 1995 by Gaia Books Limited

66 Charlotte Street   20 High Street
London W1P 1LR   Stroud, Glos GL5 1AS

First published in Great Britain in 1989
by Sidgwick & Jackson Limited, London

ISBN 1 85675 017 5

Typeset in Bembo by
Wace Publication Imaging (Sidcup),
Kent, DA14 5DT, England
Reproduction by Craft Print Pte
Printed and bound in Singapore by Craft
Print Pte
10 9 8 7 6 5 4 3 2 1

Publisher's acknowledgements
Gaia would like to extend special thanks
to the following: Dr Richard Donze,
Lesley Gilbert, The International
Cheese Centre, Georgina Wheeler, and
Table Props Hire Ltd.

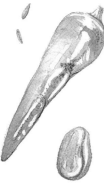
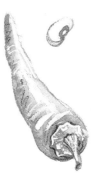

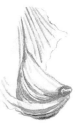

How to use this book

Chapter 1 (**A healthy diet**) explains how to choose food to give you the best possible balance of nutrients. *The basic healthy diet* (pp. 12-13) gives a breakdown of necessary nutrients and is referred to throughout the book. The rest of the chapter deals with the special dietary needs of pregnancy, breast feeding, the menopause, and gives information about processing food, and growing herbs. Chapter 2 (**The common ailments**) lists the ailments in alphabetical order, telling you how to prevent or cure through diet. Chapter 3 (**The special diets**) gives advice if you need to change your diet more dramatically.

Note   You should not use this book for self-diagnosis. Always consult a qualified practitioner if you are in doubt about a condition, and observe the instructions and cautions given in the book. The author and publishers cannot accept responsibility for changes in product ingredients, undiscovered hazards of foods or herbs, or any adverse health effects.

Glossary

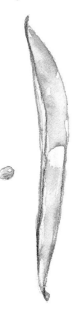

"Culprit" food   A food containing substances (nutrients, additives, etc.) to which you are sensitive.

"Empty" calories   The nutritional contribution of refined carbohydrates, or of polyunsaturated fats that have lost their essential fatty acids. These foods supply many calories, but few nutrients in their original state.

Essential fatty acids   Unsaturated fatty acids that are vital to our well-being and cannot be made in the body. They are spoilt by overheating, especially if mixed with saturated fats and by hydrogenation.

Nutrient-dense   Foods packed with essential nutrients.

Refined foods   Foods that have been processed to remove their fibre. In the refining, vitamins, fibre, and minerals are sacrificed.

Westernized diet   A diet based on large amounts of "empty" calories and animal protein, and sometimes lacking certain minerals and vitamins, essential fatty acids, and fibre.

Contents

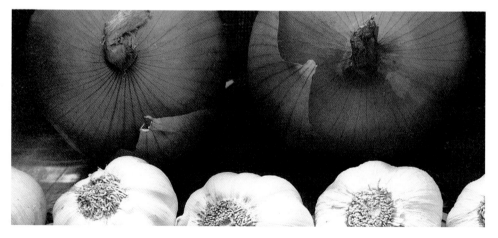

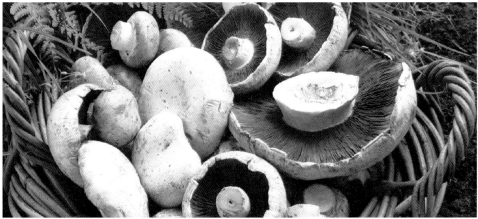

THE SPECIAL DIETS 79

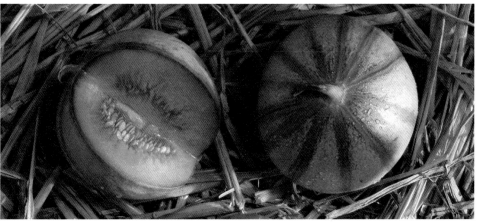

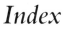

Introduction

Sages and physicians in ancient times were well aware of the strong links between food and health, but the coming of modern drug- and technology-based medicine has meant that centuries of such nutritional wisdom have evaporated almost overnight. There has been an explosion of commercial food processing, and at the same time our home and work lives have become increasingly divorced. We are no longer much involved with our food. We are opting out of preparing food in favour of using convenience foods, which are cleaned, refined, cut up, mixed, preserved, flavoured, and cooked in factories by people who have no physical or emotional connection with us. Few people grow their own fruit and vegetables, and even fewer tend their own livestock.

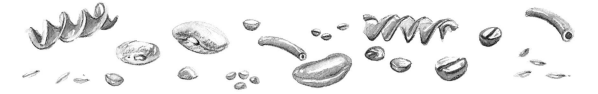

We are witnessing an unprecedented change in eating habits in affluent westernized countries, and developing countries are following suit. The average person eats a diet extraordinarily high in saturated fats, refined sugar and cereal, meat and other animal products, and commercially processed food, and surprisingly low in fresh – and raw – fruit and vegetables. No longer do we save our valuable sweet and fatty foods, and laboriously sifted flour, for feasts and festivals. Today, feasting happens every day and it has unexpectedly brought us a great deal of ill health. While more than half the world starves, the rest of us gorge. It is a paradox that nutritional deficiencies are common in the overfed. They eat too much rich, sweet, but often nutrient-poor food, and often not enough nutrient-rich staples. Nutritional deprivation through the overconsumption of high-priced, feast-time foods means that our diet is thoroughly unbalanced. As a result our health suffers.

Healthy people constantly react and adapt to the various stresses in their lives. One way of aiding these homeostatic mechanisms is by eating a healthy diet geared to age and activity, and to the special requirements of pregnancy or breastfeeding, as well as to the weather, season, time of day, and personal taste. Another is to alter the diet according to personal health and inclination, and learn to use food as a medicine when helpful. It's important to listen to the messages from the mind and body, and to become more sensitive to their needs. Continually ignored messages lead to vague symptoms of ill health. Eventually overt illness results.

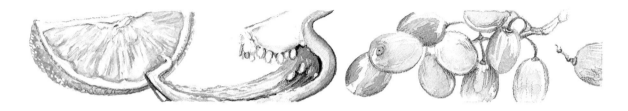

Taking responsibility

Perhaps before long we will relearn what the ancients knew – that our food can be a source of goodness and energy far beyond its calorie and biochemical content. We can alter the vibrant, dynamic, free-flowing energy that keeps us well by the food we eat. The energy the East knows as prana or Chi – the life force – is present in food more or less, depending on its quality and freshness. Good food is a vital source of wellbeing. When our vitality is blocked by a poor diet we feel unwell, lethargic, and at a low ebb. Our energy seeps out of us and we lose our zest for life. Our food is intimately linked with our vitality and with our feelings toward ourselves, others, our planet, and the source of our spiritual strength. Yet we have grown to think of it purely as a physical fuel and have lost any sense of respect for it.

Changing our diet offers us a whole new way of being. We can use our food to look after, love, restore, and heal ourselves and others. Good food offers us the chance of better physical, emotional, social, and spiritual health. Our health is far too important to be left to scientists and other "experts". We can start taking more responsibility for our wellbeing now, and our choice of the food we eat is one of the most important ways in which to do this.

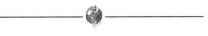

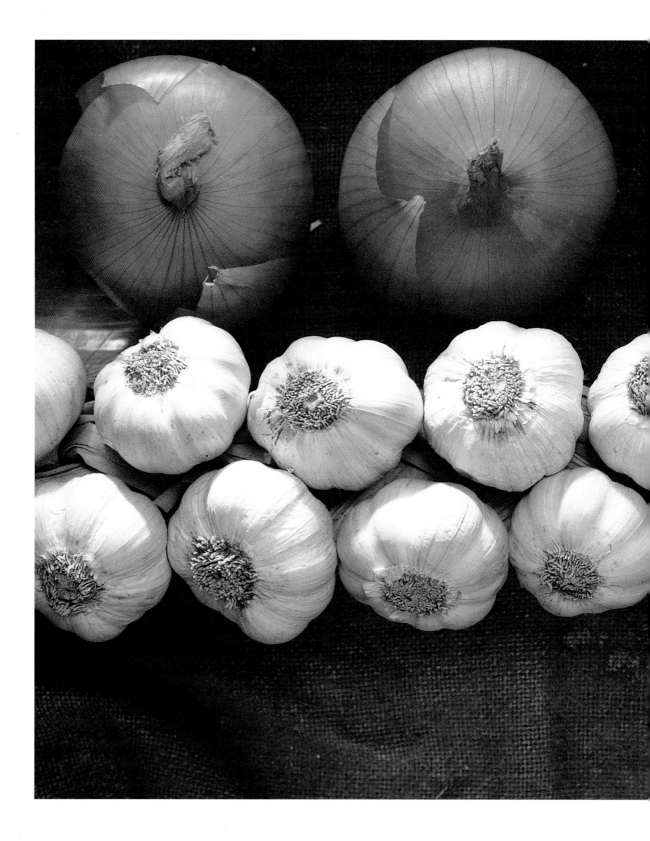

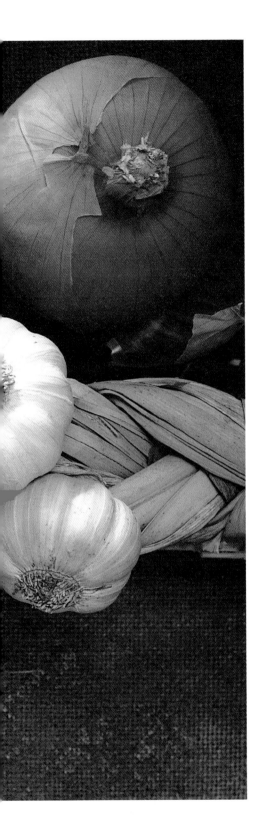

A HEALTHY DIET

The food you eat reflects your beliefs about yourself, your spiritual being, the people important to you, and the world. You can change your diet to communicate your wish for a healthier self and society.

Take a delight in everything you eat and drink throughout the day. A variety of whole cereal grains, natural rice, beans in all their hues, peas, lentils, chickpeas, nuts of different shapes, colourful fruits, the fascinating array of roots, stems, leaves, flowers, and seeds of vegetables in their myriad forms and textures, gives you endless choice. Herbs and spices add subtle sensuality. If you like meat, use it as an interesting, flavour-ful addition, feasting on it only occasionally. If you eat a diet based on whole foods, thoughtfully prepared, you will almost certainly receive all the goodness you need and the best combination of nutrients. There is usually no need for nutritional supplements. All most people need is good food – not bad food plus pills. This chapter helps guide your choice of food to nourish you more fully, both to meet normal needs and to cope with special circumstances such as pregnancy or breast feeding. It also gives information on food preparation and growing herbs.

The basic healthy diet

The main components of a basic healthy diet are: proteins, fats, carbohydrates, minerals, vitamins, and fibre. Most whole foods contain many nutrients in varying proportions, so a variety of foods will give you a good balance. To eat well and feel healthy, choose whole, fresh, or carefully processed foods, and favour those of vegetable origin.

The food groups
(See **Foods, nutrients, and ailments** *on pages 80 to 82 for examples of foods rich in essential fatty acids, fibre, minerals, and vitamins.)*

Carbohydrates and fibre Starches and sugars are in grains, fruits, pulses (peas and beans), nuts, vegetables, and milk. Starch-rich foods (whole grains, root vegetables, pulses, bananas) should form over a third of your calories. Fibre keeps the bowel healthy and protects against high cholesterol levels, certain cancers, gallstones, and obesity.

Fats provide insulation, build cells and facilitate metabolism. They are made of saturated, polyunsaturated, and mono-unsaturated fatty acids. A variety of foods provides a good balance. Animal fats and hard margarines contain more saturated fatty acids than do soft vegetable fats and oils. Essential fatty acids are unsaturated fats essential for healthy skin, circulation, bone, brain, and nerves. They are used for cell membrane metabolism and to make prostaglandins and other substances necessary to control blood clotting and inflammation.

Proteins contain amino acids (see p. 15) – used to build and repair cells and regulate metabolism. All fruits and vegetables contain some protein. Good sources are peas, beans, lentils, grains, nuts, seeds, sprouted seeds, and potatoes. Animal proteins are milk, yogurt, cheese, meat, eggs, and fish.

Minerals build and maintain bones and teeth, control the composition of body fluids and cells, and release energy. A variety of foods gives the minerals you need.

Vitamins are vital for normal body chemistry. They all come from food, but vitamin D is also produced by the action of daylight on skin, and vitamin K from micro-organisms in the bowel.

Eight-point plan

● *Eat plenty of fibre. Pulses, whole grains, foods made with wholegrain flour (such as wholegrain bread), and fruit and vegetables give you the benefit of fibre as well as its associated essential fatty acids, minerals, and vitamins. Grains are better only coarsely ground.*

● *Eat plenty of fresh fruit and vegetables, especially green leafy ones. These give the vitamins, flavonoids, minerals, essential fatty acids, and fibre you need. Peel fruit as little as possible (peel and pith are nutrient-rich). Cook vegetables lightly by steaming or stir-frying, and eat some raw daily to benefit from their hormones and enzymes.*

● *Cut down your fat intake (especially saturated fat – see pp. 83-5). Choose fish, offal (organ meat), game, poultry, whole grains, pulses, nuts and seeds, or sprouted seeds, rather than red meat and cheese.*

● *Cut down your sugar intake. Use sugar as a flavouring rather than as a food. Avoid cakes, sweets, chocolates, biscuits, puddings, ice cream, jam, fruits canned in syrup, soft drinks, sugar in tea and coffee, and milk shakes.*

● *Cut down your salt intake. Instead of adding salt to your food use herbs, spices, fresh ginger, horseradish, garlic, lemon juice, tomato purée, vinegar, soy sauce, vegetable stock, yeast extract, chutney, and other flavourings.*

● *Cut down your consumption of processed food to avoid the "empty calories" of saturated fats, added sugar, refined cereal grains, and additives.*

● *Drink only moderate amounts of alcohol.*

● *If you are overweight, exercise more and consume the amount of food and drink that will enable you to reach and keep to your optimal body weight.*

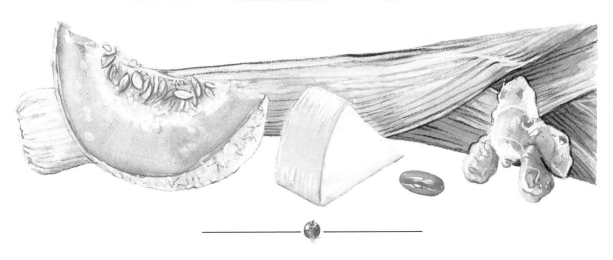

Pregnancy and breast feeding

Before you conceive it is important to eat well and be reasonably fit. *The basic healthy diet (pp.12-13)* ensures you start pregnancy with good stores of nutrients and a daily supplement of folic acid is helpful. Many find they eat much the same when pregnant as before because they exercise less, so energy requirements remain fairly constant. Also, the body probably uses food more efficiently. If your appetite is larger than before, then the extra food should be nutritious and not

You and your baby need: good supplies of protein, vitamin A, thiamine, riboflavin, niacin, vitamins B6 and B12, folic acid, vitamins C, D, and E, calcium, magnesium, zinc, iron, iodine, phosphorus, essential fatty acids, and twice as much folic acid as usual.

"empty" calories. Weight gain varies widely – from 7-18kg (15-40lb) – from woman to woman. No one is sure how much alcohol, if any, is safe during pregnancy, but alcoholic binges are foolish. If you are vegetarian, check you are eating enough foods rich in iron, zinc, and vitamin B12.

Diet during breast feeding

If you do not eat well when you are breast feeding, your own body may suffer (as stored nutrients pass to the baby) and you may not produce enough milk. To nourish both of you, you need a nutritious diet (see *the basic health diet*), and about 300-600 extra nutrient-rich calories on top of this each day. Your "junk food margin" does not increase, so avoid "empty" calories. The bigger the baby, the more milk is needed, and the more you will have to eat to produce it.

The menopause

If you eat a *basic healthy diet* you enter your menopause with an advantage. This diet continues to protect against osteoporosis and other problems associated with changing hormone

levels, especially if you take enough exercise and fresh air. As you get older, your "junk food margin" lessens, so it is even more important to eat high-quality, nutritious food.

Mixed and vegetarian diets?

Vegetarians have less heart disease, cancer, digestive problems and osteoporosis than meat-eaters. This is probably because they eat more protective foods, which include vegetables, fruit, nuts, seeds, wholegrains, pulses and legumes. You can safely eat meat, fish, eggs and dairy food in moderation, but excessive amounts may be risky. Unlike vegetable protein, too much of this sulphur-laced protein leaches calcium from bones, encouraging osteoporosis and kidney disease.

Also, red meat and dairy food contain a lot of saturated fat, and too much of this in the diet makes heart disease and some cancers more likely.

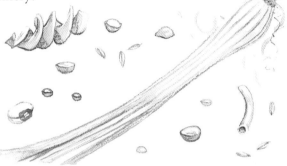

Food processing

Almost all foods are processed in some way before you eat them. Some nutrients, such as vitamins B, C, and E, and certain minerals are lost to a varying degree during processing. Losses due to home cooking can be greater than those resulting from factory processing. It is important to reduce these losses as much as you can (especially when cooking for the very young, the pregnant, the elderly, the sick, and those with a poor appetite).

Some processing is essential for most foods. Grains, for example, need to be cooked unless allowed to sprout. Before you cook a food you need to prepare it, perhaps by cutting or peeling, both of which can lead to nutrient loss. Rough handling and slicing or shredding reduce the vitamin C content. Do not prepare foods until immediately before you eat or cook them – an enzyme that destroys vitamin C is released by cutting, but is inactivated by heat. Many organically grown fruits and vegetables are better eaten with their peel or outside leaves on because these contain high concentrations of some vitamins and minerals, and fibre.

There are many methods of preserving food, including drying, heating, freezing, chilling, fermenting, smoking, bottling in syrup, canning in syrup or saline, pasteurizing, and irradiating.

Some methods have disadvantages. Dehydrating potatoes to make instant potato, for example, destroys most of their vitamin C. Blanching vegetables before freezing leads to a 25% loss of vitamin C, with more lost later during cooking. Canning destroys 50% of the folic acid in food and some of the vitamins B6 and C. Pasteurizing removes 7% of the vitamin B12 in milk and ultra-heat treatment 20%. Drying milk leads to losses of vitamin B6. Freezing fried foods destroys vitamin E.

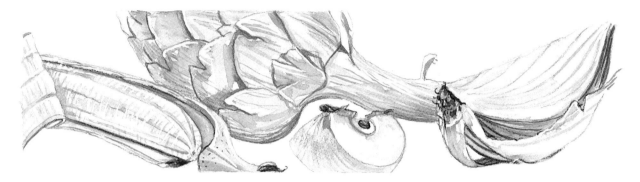

Cooking methods

To retain vitamins in your food:

Vitamin A Avoid cooking at high temperatures – this destroys some of the vitamin by oxidation.

B vitamins Avoid washing, soaking, or boiling, as B vitamins are water soluble and easily lost. Even brief boiling destroys up to a third of vitamin B12 and half the folic acid.

Vitamin C This vitamin is water soluble and heat sensitive.

To reduce losses:
- Use as little water as possible.
- Add food to rapidly boiling water.
- Cover the pan.
- Do not add sodium bicarbonate.
- Avoid using copper pans.
- Use cooking water for soups, sauces, and gravies.
- Serve and eat promptly.

Vitamin E Avoid frying or baking as up to 50% is lost.

Proteins Avoid overheating as this destroys some amino acids.

Fats Heating fats to high temperatures destroys essential fatty acids and can make them indigestible, and even possibly cancer-inducing. Avoid reusing fat; frequent deep-frying; and frying for long periods.

Herbs

You can buy herbal teas, and fresh and dried herbs from many health food stores and supermarkets. Better still, grow your own herbs. You can grow most of the ones mentioned in this book in temperate climates. A few flourish only in hot climates.

Growing herbs at home

To grow herbs in a window box, cover the base with a layer of broken clay pots; add 5cm (2in) of sand; then add potting compost or soil; and cover with a peat mulch. Some herbs, such as mint, borage, and meadowsweet, tolerate full shade. Others, such as sage, chervil, lemon balm, and parsley, like a little sun. A sunny position is essential for garlic, chamomile, feverfew, thyme, rosemary, lavender, dill, and marjoram. If you are growing herbs in pots, put those that like sun by an open sunny window, or outside, in summer. All herbs benefit from regular feeds in the growing season.

How to harvest and store herbs

Cut stems on a warm, dry day. Handle gently to avoid bruising. Spread them out to dry on a layer of muslin stretched over a box in a warm, airy place indoors. Turn the herbs every day until quite dry then store in a dark glass jar. Some herbs freeze well. Tie in bunches, and blanch for 1 minute. Chill in cold water, then hang to dry. Freeze in plastic bags.

How to make herbal tea

Use one teaspoonful of dried or two teaspoonsful of fresh herbs to a pint of boiling water. Infuse for up to 5 minutes (lemon balm needs 15 minutes). Strain before drinking. If you use seeds or berries, soak until they start to swell, then drain first.

WARNING

Chamomile tea If you are allergic to chrysanthemums, asters, ragweed, goldenrod, or marigolds, you may also be allergic to chamomile. You may feel sick if it is strong.

Valerian tea This tea contains potent chemicals. Drink commercially available tea in moderation only. Consult a medical herbalist about strong preparations.

Lime-flower tea Make sure fresh lime flowers are not wilting.

Feverfew tea Avoid in pregnancy.

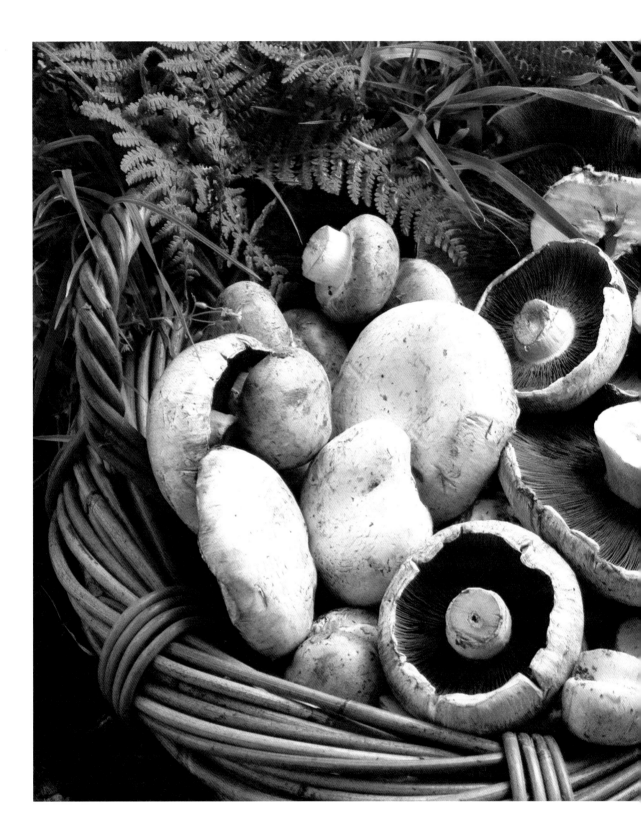

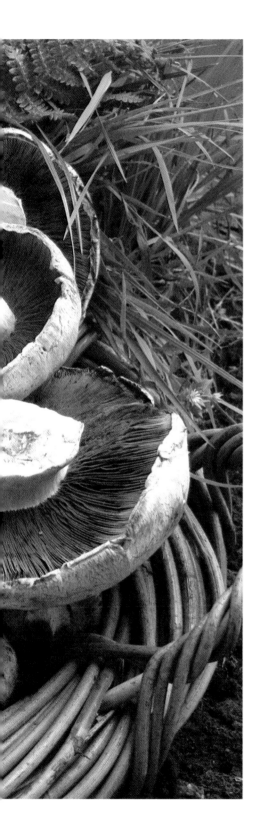

THE COMMON AILMENTS

The language of our relationship with food may not be readily apparent, but it is trying to say something important. Many people suffer from hidden emotions such as fear, anger, and sadness, from unexpressed needs for love, comfort, security, control and rewards, and from powerful drives towards self-destruction. Only by making sense of the messages coming across in their lifestyles and in their relationship to food can they hope to recognize what is going on and meet their needs in more constructive ways.

Our diet and the way we eat resonates with our attitudes to living together, to celebration, to sex, and to our spiritual lives. Our feast days are often little different to ordinary days. Our lust for too much meat and sweet, fatty, over-processed foods is similar to our craving for the material things of this world. Never before have so many people been so unaware of their spiritual dimension.

Ancient wisdom acknowledges that we can influence how we feel physically, emotionally, intellectually, and spiritually by what we eat. Ayurvedic medicine, for example, tailors the diet to the individual, taking into account constitution, body type, taste, season, time of day, food combinations, and whether food is heavy or light, heat- or cold-producing, liquid or solid, and raw or cooked. Shintoism points to our one-ness with nature, the importance of the colours and shapes of foods, and the sacredness of food as we grow, prepare, serve, and eat it. Macrobiotics recommends a balanced diet including whole grains, pulses, seeds, vegetables, and only small amounts of very "yin" foods (sugar, alcohol, tea, and coffee) and very "yang" foods (meat, eggs, cheese, and salt). Despite knowing this, the degree of westernized people's unsophistication over how food affects the body, mind, and spirit is astonishing.

The cost of unhealthy eating

However well we look after ourselves, we may become ill. But we can accept illness in a positive, healthy way by continuing to take heed of the signals from our bodies and minds. Obesity, heart attacks, strokes, diabetes, gallstones, diverticular disease, and bowel and breast cancer can all be linked with what we eat. Such disorders are to some extent preventable. In the US three out of four people are estimated to die from diet-related diseases, and it is thought that up to 35 per cent of cancers could be prevented. Experts agree on the changes we need in our diet. While no dietary change is a panacea, poor eating habits can adversely affect every condition. They also tend to echo down the generations as children often eat as adults what they were brought up to eat. Even rich countries can no longer afford the increasing costs of a health care system based on drugs and technology. Ill health costs individuals and families dearly and exerts a heavy toll on nations, too.

We live in an age strongly influenced by market forces. Farmers, preferring a quick return on their investment, opt for factory farming and the often excessive use of agrichemicals. These methods may produce more food, but they also influence its quality. The food industry makes more money from selling high-priced, "technological" foods than from staples. Advertisements lead us to crave the very foods that allay our hunger for more healthy fare. And there is little money allocated to promote whole foods. Government policy is easily swayed by the power of vested commercial interest and professional lobbies. Rather than farmers being encouraged to produce organically grown food, or more money being spent on health education, we are blamed for our choice of food.

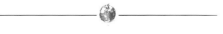

We need to look more deeply at what is happening. Perhaps our self-esteem is so low that we no longer believe we deserve to be nourished well and to take thoughtful, loving care over our food. Food is like love. We need the right amounts of both if we are to grow up healthy. Without food or love we die, and with the wrong sort we fail to thrive. But there is another connection. Our attitude to food is based on our experience of being loved and our ability to love ourselves and others. Many often unconscious emotions are symbolized by what we eat and the way we eat it. People sometimes act out their emotions by becoming anorexic or bulimic.

This chapter lists the most common ailments and illnesses. Each entry first describes how to prevent and treat the ailment by adjusting your diet, and then recommends specific foods. If you cannot find an entry for your ailment, refer to the index. Foods and nutrients are mentioned constantly, so you should turn to **The basic healthy diet** on pages 12 and 13 and the **Foods, nutrients, and ailments** chart on pages 80 to 82 for further information. At the end of each entry is a summary of foods and/or nutrients you should either increase (▲) or decrease (▼) – this advice presupposes that you are already eating the basic healthy diet. To gain maximum benefit from the summary, first read the entire entry to determine whether the advice applies to you. All the nutrients recommended (vitamin C, for instance) are intended to be eaten in the form of foods high in that nutrient (oranges, for instance) and NOT as supplements. The recommendations are for when you are unwell. When you are better, the basic healthy diet will help keep you that way. When necessary, liaise with your doctor over the cause and treatment of your ailment. Ailments in italics within each entry indicate an entry elsewhere in the chapter.

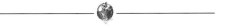

Acid reflux (heartburn)

Acid reflux is more likely if your stomach is too full; if you swallow excess air, or eat wind-producing (gas-producing) foods; if your diet is high in refined carbohydrates; if you drink a large amount of alcohol; or if you chew inadequately. If you are overweight you are more likely to suffer because being fat can affect the action of the valve at the lower end of the gullet, and you are more at risk if the valve has been weakened by straining to pass bowel motions.

Diet Peppermint or meadowsweet tea may help. You can prevent it by avoiding large meals, fatty foods, refined carbohydrates, cocoa, strong coffee or tea, and alcohol within three hours of bed. If you do drink alcohol, eat something with it. Eat slowly and chew well to prepare food for further digestion. Alter your diet to prevent or cure *constipation* and lose weight, if necessary. (See **The basic healthy diet** pp. 12-13, **Foods, nutrients, and ailments** pp. 80-2, **The weight-reducing diet** pp. 87-9.)

▲ Peppermint, and meadowsweet teas.

▼ Fats; refined carbohydrates (including added sugar); coffee, tea, cocoa, alcohol.

Acne

In acne there is inflammation around the sebaceous glands, with infection in their ducts, increased production of sebum, and melanin pigmentation of the sebum that lies stagnating in the ducts (blackheads). The level of vitamin A in your blood will be lower than normal, even though you may think you are getting enough in your diet. Researchers have found large amounts of vitamin A in blackheads themselves, indicating that sufferers may need more vitamin A in their diet to replace this loss. Acne is a very common complaint and is associated with the diet of westernized countries, where up to 80 per cent of teenagers have the symptoms.

Diet If you eat *the basic healthy diet*, which is low in refined carbohydrates and saturated fats (including whole-milk dairy foods), and high in fibre and essential fatty acids, you have a better chance of preventing acne. Avoid refined sugar, as this reduces the body's vitamin A level. Choose vegetable rather than animal proteins. Eat more foods containing zinc, selenium, essential fatty acids and vitamins A, B6, C, and E, and more raw fruits and vegetables (especially green leafy vegetables and those containing vitamin A). It may help to supplement these with fresh juices made

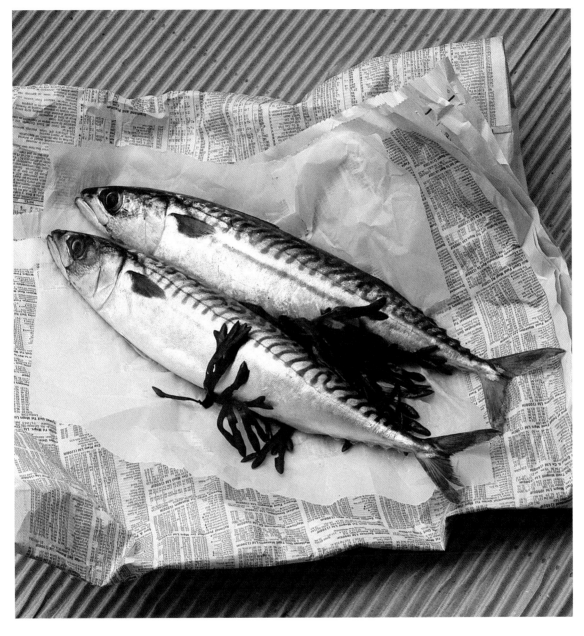

Mackerel is high in essential "omega 3" fatty acids. Two of these acids, EPA and DMA, make red cells more supple and blood less sticky, and also help maintain a healthy balance of low- and high-density lipoproteins (LDL and MDL cholesterol) in the blood. Mackerel is also rich in protein and vitamins B and D.

from beetroot or carrots. Crushed, raw garlic (about three cloves a day) is also worth trying. Once your acne has begun to improve you should stick to this eating plan to prevent recurrences. Some people find that certain foods, such as chocolate, make acne worse, but this has not yet been confirmed by medical research. Chocolate may affect women at a particular point in their menstrual cycle only, so observing its effects at other times is useless. If you think foods affect your skin, record what you eat, when you menstruate, and when you have acne, to pinpoint "culprit" foods. (See **The basic healthy diet** pp. 12-13, **Foods, nutrients, and ailments** pp. 80-2, **The exclusion diet** pp. 91-3.)

▲ Raw vegetables (especially green leafy ones and garlic); essential fatty acids; vitamins A, B6, C, and E; zinc.

▼ Refined carbohydrates (especially added sugar); "culprit" foods.

Ageing

Some people age faster than others and run a greater risk of suffering from disorders such as osteoporosis, *diverticular disease*, *arterial disease*, and senile *confusion*. You can prevent many of these problems by eating *the basic healthy diet* in youth and middle age as well as in later years. As you grow older you need less food, but the digestion and absorption of nutrients become less efficient so its best to avoid too many "empty calories".

Diet Help prevent premature ageing by eating a *basic healthy diet* containing plenty of raw fruit and vegetables, including garlic, and avoid refined carbohydrates and excessive alcohol. Proteins should form only about 13 per cent of your calorie intake. Lose excess weight because slim yet well-nourished people tend to age more slowly and have fewer ailments. Make sure you are getting enough vitamins A, niacin, C, and E, selenium, zinc, copper, and manganese, particularly if you are unwell. It is vital to consume enough essential fatty acids together with the magnesium, zinc, and vitamin B6 you need to metabolize them. Vitamin C, flavonoids, and zinc all help keep skin supple. (See **The basic healthy diet** pp. 12-13, **Foods, nutrients, and ailments** pp. 80-2, **The weight-reducing diet** pp. 87-9.)

▲ Raw vegetables and fruit; vitamins A, niacin, B6, C, E; flavonoids; selenium, zinc, copper, magnesium, manganese; essential fatty acids.

▼ Excess protein; "empty" calories, excess alcohol.

Alcoholism

If you find it difficult to cope with life without consuming alcohol daily, or nearly every day, you may be becoming dependent on drink. If you have two or more drinks a day you are more likely to develop one of the alcohol-influenced disorders. These include liver and heart disorders, certain *cancers*, *gout*, *diabetes*, gastritis, chest infections, *depression*, mood swings, and mental breakdown. A "drink" is a single measure (shot) of spirits (hard liquor), a half pint (10oz) of beer, a glass (4.5oz) of wine, or a small sherry. Ask for help from Alcoholics Anonymous or another support group and set about adjusting your diet. *The basic healthy diet* makes you much less likely to crave alcohol. If you are alcohol-dependent, it helps to reduce your addiction and replaces nutrients that alcohol has either supplanted, prevented the body from absorbing or using, or flushed out in the urine.

Diet Check that you are eating plenty of raw vegetables and fruit, and cut down alcohol, or stop drinking it altogether. Alcohol contains many calories, but few useful nutrients. If you are an alcoholic you run the risk of becoming overweight and because alcohol satisfies your appetite, you may go short of vital nutrients. The more you drink, the more important it is to choose your foods wisely – your "junk food margin" is very small. Alcohol reduces the absorption and metabolic action of many nutrients, including most of the B vitamins, vitamins A and D, folic acid, calcium, phosphorus, zinc, protein, certain amino acids, essential fatty acids, and glucose, and it tends to flush magnesium out of the body in the urine. This means that it is easy to become deficient in these nutrients, and your diet should include foods rich in them. Foods rich in thiamine may help stop you craving alcohol – it is possible that this craving may represent a *food-sensitive* craving for the food from which the alcohol was fermented. You may be sensitive to yeast, too. If you think this might apply to you, test for a food sensitivity. It is probably better to avoid alcohol just before conception, and during pregnancy, and too much alcohol while breastfeeding. (See **The basic healthy diet** pp. 12-13, **Foods, nutrients, and ailments** pp. 80-2, **The exclusion diet** pp. 91-3.)

▲ Vitamins A, B, and D; folic acid; calcium, magnesium, phosphorus, zinc; protein; essential fatty acids; raw vegetables and fruits.

▼ "Empty" calories; alcohol; "culprit" foods.

Anaemia

The commonest cause of iron-deficiency anaemia in women is insufficient iron in the diet to replace menstrual losses.

Diet You can help prevent anaemia by eating *the basic healthy diet*, with a variety of fresh, raw vegetables (especially green leafy ones). The body absorbs iron from raw vegetables more easily than from cooked ones. Increase your iron-rich foods and eat plenty of vitamin C- and copper-containing foods, garlic, and onions to aid iron absorption. Do not use up too much of your calorie intake with dairy foods. Avoid coffee, tea, cola, and tannin-containing herbal teas from about one hour before meals to an hour and a half after. These reduce iron absorption and flush excess water through the kidneys, leading to a loss of some of the nutrients needed to form haemoglobin, such as magnesium, and vitamin B6. Some anaemic people make too little gastric acid. Gastric acid aids iron absorption. Carbohydrates tend to lower stomach acid, so avoid eating carbohydrates with iron-rich meat, fish, or eggs. Eat more zinc and niacin, both needed for acid production, and have some vinegar with proteins. (See **The basic healthy diet** pp. 12-13, **Foods, nutrients, and ailments** pp. 80-2.)

▲ Raw vegetables; niacin, vitamin C; iron, copper, zinc.

▼ Coffee, tea, cocoa, cola, alcohol.

Anxiety

Nutritional deficiencies or imbalances may encourage fear or panic.

Diet Keep to *the basic healthy diet*, especially when under stress. If you are feeling tense, cut added sugar from your diet and eat plenty of complex carbohydrates (wholegrain bread and pasta, potatoes, beans, peas and lentils. Don't eat meat, fish or eggs at the same time as this cancels carbohydrate's calming effect. Eating little but often helps avoid these swings. Caffeine-containing drinks can cause anxiety; as can *food sensitivity* and alcohol. If your diet is lacking calcium, magnesium, niacin or vitamin E, this may be contributing to your anxiety. Valerian, chamomile flower, lime flower, or passion flower teas have a calming effect. (See **The basic healthy diet** pp. 12-13, **Foods, nutrients, and ailments** pp. 80-2, **The exclusion diet** pp. 91-3.)

▲ Complex carbohydrates; niacin and vitamin E; calcium, magnesium; valerian, chamomile flower, lime, and passion flower teas.

▼ Added sugar; tea, coffee, cocoa, cola; "culprit" foods; alcohol.

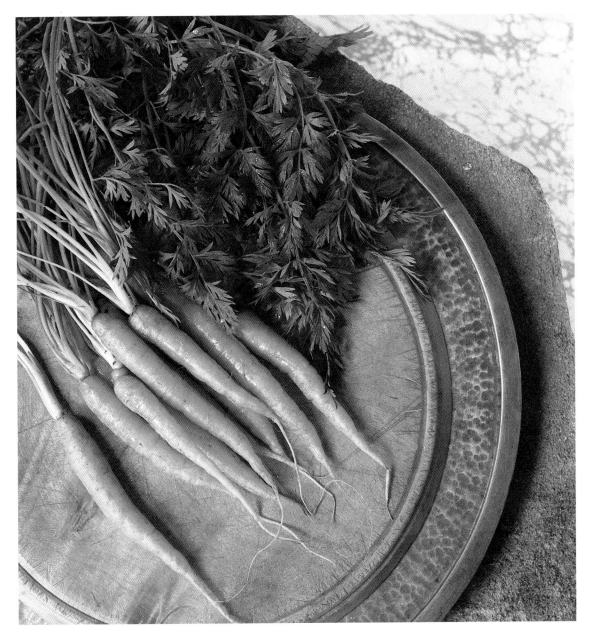

Carrots *are bursting with beta-carotene, necessary for growth and for the healthy functioning of the retina in the eye, the linings of the breathing and digestive passages, and the urinary and genital tracts. Prepare carrots by scrubbing, not scraping or peeling, since the greatest concentration of vitamins, flavonoids and minerals lie in or just below the surface.*

Appendicitis

Inflammation, and perhaps infection, of the appendix can cause abdominal pain and nausea (a "grumbling" appendix), or acute appendicitis, which needs surgery. The inflammation is provoked by the blockage of the appendix by hard-to-pass bowel motions.

Diet Help prevent appendicitis by eating the *basic healthy diet* with plenty of high-fibre foods. If you eat refined carbohydrates, help counteract their effect by taking high-fibre foods on the same day and plenty of water. *Infection* can complicate appendix inflammation, so eat more infection-fighting foods (see p.54). (See **The basic healthy diet** pp. 12-13, **Foods, nutrients, and ailments** pp. 80-2.)

▲ High-fibre foods (especially green leafy vegetables); water; infection fighting foods.

▼ Refined carbohydrates (including added sugar).

Appetite loss

The appetite is controlled by neurotransmitter chemicals in the hypothalamus. These are influenced by the blood levels of sugar, fatty acids, and hormones, which can be affected by shock, *anxiety*, *depression*, long-term illness, digestive disorders, fever, *cancer*, and a deficiency of thiamine, or pantothenic acid, or zinc. Treat the underlying cause of your appetite loss first.

Diet Try to eat frequent, small meals of foods you like and follow *the basic healthy diet*. Your "junk food margin" is low because your calorie intake is lower than normal. Check that you are eating enough foods containing vitamins, thiamine, pantothenic acid, and zinc. Teas made with fenugreek seeds, juniper berries, clover flowers, or yarrow may stimulate your appetite. (See **The basic healthy diet** pp. 12-13, **Foods, nutrients, and ailments** pp. 80-2.)

▲ Small, frequent amounts of food and drink; thiamine and pantothenic acid; zinc; fenugreek, juniper, clover, or yarrow tea.

▼ "Empty" calories.

Arterial disease

Arterial disease underlies most cardiovascular disease, including angina, poor circulation (see *Circulation problems*), leg pain on walking, *high blood pressure*, heart attacks, strokes, and sudden death. Poor diet is one of the major causes. The natural wear and tear on arteries creates tiny tears in artery linings. These normally heal quickly, but a poor diet can lead to thickened scars and stiffened, roughened walls (arteriosclerosis or "hardening of the arteries"). When the blood levels of saturated fats surge high after a fatty meal, the tears are impregnated with fats, leading to poor healing. Saturated fats adhere to the rough walls, forming fat-rich atheroma, which further weakens arteries and encourages bleeding. Blood is more likely to clot if artery walls are rough and the arteries are narrowed by atheroma. Populations with low levels of arterial disease eat less saturated fat.

It is sensible to eat a diet aimed at keeping the arteries healthy from childhood, though you can slow, prevent, or reverse further damage at any age. First, adjust your diet to prevent *high blood pressure*. Second, eat less total fat and less saturated fat (meat, dairy products, hard margarines, and soft margarines containing trans fats). Some people need to eat less cholesterol (see p.83). Third, make sure that your blood levels of saturated fats never surge too high (see below). Fourth, eat adequate amounts of the nutrients that maintain arterial elasticity, aid replacement and repair of artery lining cells, help stop blood clotting dangerously, and help keep levels of saturated fats low.

Diet If you are too heavy, lose weight. Reduce your total and saturated fat intake. This increases the proportion of unsaturated fats in your diet. You can help prevent your blood levels of saturated fats from surging too high by avoiding large amounts of saturated-fat-containing food at any one meal, and by cutting added sugar down or out. Sugar increases the absorption of fats and raises blood fat levels, and alcohol has a similar action. The liver converts both sugar and alcohol into saturated blood fats.

You can emulsify fats and lessen the tendency of the blood to clot by eating oily fish and other foods containing essential fatty acids; garlic (about three cloves daily) and onions; pineapple; ginger; avocados; and foods containing vitamins thiamine, B6, C (and possibly E), flavonoids, vegetable lecithin, and natural salicylates (see p.92). Oily fish help make certain beneficial prostaglandins, which reduce abnormal blood clotting. Lecithin regulates the blood levels of fats, emulsifies blood fats, and is an anti-coagulant; the amount and quality we absorb may vary with our diet.

Increase your fruit and vegetables (especially apples, citrus fruits, carrots and green leafy vegetables), pulses (beans and peas), oats, and foods containing calcium, chromium, copper, magnesium, zinc, selenium, silicon, vanadium, lecithin, vitamin A, niacin and fibre. If you suffer from angina, avoid heavy meals and excessive alcohol (see *Alcoholism*). However, a small amount (such as a glass of wine) half an hour before your main meal may be helpful. (See **The basic healthy diet** pp. 12-13, **Food, nutrients, and ailments** pp. 80-2, **The weight-reducing diet** pp. 87-9.)

▲ Oily fish; lecithin and essential fatty acids, raw fruit and vegetables (especially apples, citrus fruit and green leafy vegetables), garlic, onions, pulses, oats, avocados, pineapple, ginger; vitamins A, B6, C, and E, thiamine, niacin, flavonoids; fibre; natural salicylates; calcium, chromium, copper, magnesium, zinc, selenium, silicon, vanadium.

▼ Total fats; saturated fats; cholesterol; added sugar; excessive alcohol.

Arthritis

Arthritis is inflammation in a joint and the main types are osteoarthritis, rheumatoid arthritis, and *gout*. You can sometimes influence osteoarthritis by diet. It is more likely if you are overweight because of wear and tear on weight-bearing joints. Rheumatoid arthritis affects the whole body and may be eased by diet. Both osteoarthritis and rheumatoid arthritis are more common in westernized countries. Aluminium poisoning from cookware, bleached flour, or possibly from drinking water in some areas can cause arthritis.

Diet For osteoarthritis, reduce both total fats and saturated fats and lose weight (if necessary). Eat more foods rich in vitamins A, B, C, and E, which tend to reduce inflammation, and eat adequate amounts of calcium, iron, zinc, copper, selenium, manganese and essential fatty acids. Tomatoes, potatoes, peppers, and aubergines (eggplants) may make arthritis worse.

For rheumatoid arthritis there are four ways you can adjust your diet. The first is to eat more oily fish, fruit and vegetables (especially raw, green leafy), foods rich in zinc, copper, calcium, potassium, manganese, selenium, vitamins A, B (especially pantothenic acid and B6), C, and E, flavonoids, and pineapple, and less acid-producing food (see pp. 80-2). A *semi-fast diet* one day a week may help. Try this for several months before moving on to the second diet if necessary. The second way is to eat a diet based on fish, brown rice, cooked and raw vegetables, and fruit. (This diet should be supervised by your doctor or dietician.) The third way is to try *the exclusion diet* for three weeks. Common "culprit" foods are, in order, cereals, red meat, sugar, saturated fats, salt, coffee, dairy foods, and potatoes. The fourth way is to eat animal protein and carbohydrate at different times. Try adding feverfew leaves to salads to help reduce the pain, but do not eat them for more than 14 consecutive days. Nettle or coriander tea may help. (See **The basic healthy diet** pp. 12-13, **Foods, nutrients, and ailments** pp. 80-2, **The weight-reducing diet** pp. 87-9, **The semi-fast diet** p. 90, **The exclusion diet** pp. 91-3.)

▲ (For osteoarthritis) vitamins A, B, C and E; calcium, iron, copper, selenium, manganese, zinc; feverfew leaves; nettle or coriander tea. (For rheumatoid arthritis) vegetables and fruit; oily fish; vitamins A, B, C, and E, flavonoids; zinc, copper, calcium, potassium, manganese, selenium; essential fatty acids; pineapple; feverfew leaves; nettle or coriander tea.

▼ (For osteoarthritis) saturated fats; "culprit" foods. (For rheumatoid arthritis) acid-producing foods; "culprit" foods.

Bad breath

Bad breath can be a sign of poor oral hygiene; of the consumption of foods of animal origin, garlic, raw onions, or alcohol; and of tooth decay, gum disease, respiratory infections, fasting, or *food sensitivity*. Some people produce insufficient gastric acid, which can lead to the fermentation of food and unpleasant gases. Adding vinegar to meat, fish and eggs may help, as may niacin-containing foods .Bad breath may be associated with *anaemia*, osteoporosis, *diabetes*, rheumatoid *arthritis, ageing, candidiasis*, and fever.

Diet　Eat *the basic healthy diet*, with plenty of green leafy vegetables. Sometimes a diet high in refined carbohydrates, coffee, and cows' milk produces bad breath. Chewing parsley counteracts the smell of garlic or onions, while chewing fennel, dill or caraway seeds, or aniseed disguises bad breath. (See **The basic healthy diet** pp. 12-13, **Foods, nutrients, and ailments** pp. 80-2.)

▲ Green leafy vegetables; niacin.

▼ Refined carbohydrates; coffee; cows' milk; "culprit" foods.

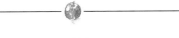

Bed-wetting

Sometimes bed-wetting is influenced by the diet.

Diet   Avoid overeating, drink only water after lunch, and only small drinks before bed. Caffeine-containing drinks increase urine output. Some people are sensitive to one or more foods (see *Food sensitivity*). Try cutting out food colourings first – if this fails try to pinpoint other "culprit" foods. Foods containing oxalate, such as spinach, strawberries, and rhubarb, can lead to an increased frequency of passing urine and bed-wetting, so restrict these foods to the mornings, or eat them with calcium-rich foods. (See **The basic healthy diet** pp. 12-13, **Foods, nutrients, and ailments** pp. 80-2, **The exclusion diet** pp. 91-3.)

▼ Fluids from lunchtime onward, especially flavoured drinks, tea, coffee, cocoa, and cola; food colourings; oxalates, unless accompanied by calcium; "culprit" foods.

Behaviour and learning problems

The diet is one factor affecting behaviour and the ability to learn.

Diet   Cut down on refined carbohydrates. Avoid added sugar as a regular part of the diet, particularly unaccompanied by protein or dietary fibre. Check whether the child is anaemic (because a deficiency of iron is fairly common) and if so, give more iron-containing foods. It is important to treat *anaemia* because an iron-deficient child is more likely to absorb environmental lead, which in itself can produce difficulties. Make sure that there are sufficient calcium and magnesium-containing foods in the diet because these are natural tranquillizers and a deficiency may cause behaviour and learning problems. Other deficiencies to watch out for are of zinc, thiamine and vitamin B6, and essential fatty acids. Too much aluminium, possibly from cooking in aluminium pans, from bleached flour, and from high levels in drinking water can lead to hyperactivity and other behaviour problems. Some children are sensitive to wheat, dairy foods, citrus fruits, eggs, chocolate, and foods containing natural salicylates (see p.92), while some preservatives and colourings affect a few children. Try to pinpoint "culprit" foods. (See **The basic healthy diet** pp. 12-13, **Foods, nutrients, and ailments** pp. 80-2, **The exclusion diet** pp. 91-3.)

▲ Essential fatty acids; thiamine and vitamin B6; calcium, iron, magnesium, zinc.

▼ Refined carbohydrates; "culprit" foods; aluminium.

Breast-feeding problems

The commonest breast-feeding problem is insufficient milk and the commonest cause is not feeding often enough or for long enough. If you are not eating well you still produce milk, and the milk has first call on the nutrients in your diet. Continued malnourishment means you will develop nutrient deficiencies; eventually the milk supply will fall and may lack some of the vital nutrients. Several dietary measures may help. You may be able to help a blocked duct and colic by adjusting your diet.

Diet To make more milk, eat a basic healthy breast-feeding diet (see p. 14) and avoid "empty calories". Eat something before or after each feed, and spread your calorie intake throughout the day. A moderate amount of traditionally brewed beer improves the milk supply by increasing prolactin levels, though this does not apply to other forms of alcohol (and excess alcohol can interfere with the let-down reflex). Useful herbal teas include those made from borage, dill, raspberry leaf, and fenugreek or caraway seed. Nettle juice, fennel, and celery may help, as may crushed fenugreek seeds. For a blocked duct eat less saturated fat, and more vegetable lecithin and essential fatty acids. For colic, eat well and spread your calorie intake – it may help not to eat large amounts of any one food at once. Cut caffeine-containing drinks down or out. Some babies react to traces of foods in the milk – common "culprits" are onions, alcohol, cabbage, and fruit. (See **The basic healthy diet** pp. 12-13, **Foods, nutrients, and ailments** pp. 80-2.)

▲ (For insufficient milk) beer; borage, dill, or raspberry leaf teas; fenugreek, and caraway seeds; nettle juice; fennel, celery. (For blocked duct) lecithin and essential fatty acids.

▼ (For insufficient milk) "empty" calories; excessive alcohol. (For blocked duct) saturated fat. (For colic) tea, coffee, cocoa, cola; "culprit" foods.

Breast problems

Many women in westernized countries suffer from breast disorders and adjusting the diet can be very helpful.

Diet Lose weight if necessary, because breast problems are more common in overweight women. *The basic healthy diet* helps prevent breast problems. It may help to reduce your intake of saturated fats (especially animal fats) in relation to unsaturated fats still further. Oily fish are thought to be useful. Avoid caffeine-containing

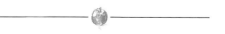

drinks. Sometimes a *food sensitivity* makes breast disease worse – if you think this may be a problem, try to find your "culprit" foods. *The low-salt diet* may help if your breast tenderness is caused by fluid retention. If your diet has been poor recently, eat more foods containing magnesium, zinc, and vitamins A, B (especially B6), and E. (See **The basic healthy diet** pp. 12-13, **Foods, nutrients, and ailments** pp. 80-2, **The low-salt diet** p. 86, **The weight-reducing diet** pp. 87-9, **The exclusion diet** pp. 91-3.)

▲ Oily fish; vitamins A, B (especially B6), E; magnesium, zinc.

▼ Saturated fat (especially animal fat); salt; "culprit" foods; tea, coffee, cocoa, cola.

Cancer

Altering your diet can help prevent or even cure some cancers. Vegetarians have less cancer than meat-eaters, perhaps not because meat is "bad" but because fruit and vegetables are "good".

Diet The ideal diet for prevention is *the basic healthy diet*. There are many reasons for this. First, it is low in fat and some cancers are more likely if you eat too much fat, especially saturated fat, and too many calories. *Obesity* is linked with an increased risk of cancer of the breast, gallbladder, and uterus, and even being 5 per cent overweight increases this risk a little. A diet high in saturated fat leads to an increased risk of cancer of the large bowel. A high-fat diet means more bile must be made; bile is altered by bacteria in the gut and may release carcinogens as a result. When you eat a lot of saturated fat, more oestrogens are manufactured in the bowel and these are associated with a higher risk of breast cancer.

Second, *the basic healthy diet* is high in fibre and insufficient dietary fibre seems to promote cancer of the colon. This may be because fibre actively protects you from cancer, or it may be simply because a diet too low in fibre tends to be too high in fat, too. Women with a history of *constipation* have an increased risk of breast cancer.

Third, *the basic healthy diet* provides plenty of foods containing vitamin A (which lowers the risk of cancer of the throat, oesophagus, lung, stomach, large bowel, bladder, and prostate); vitamin C (associated with a lower risk of cancer of the oesophagus); vitamin E (which may reduce the risk of cancer by protecting fats from going rancid – associated with higher levels of carcinogens); vitamin B6 (which may reduce the risk of cancer of the

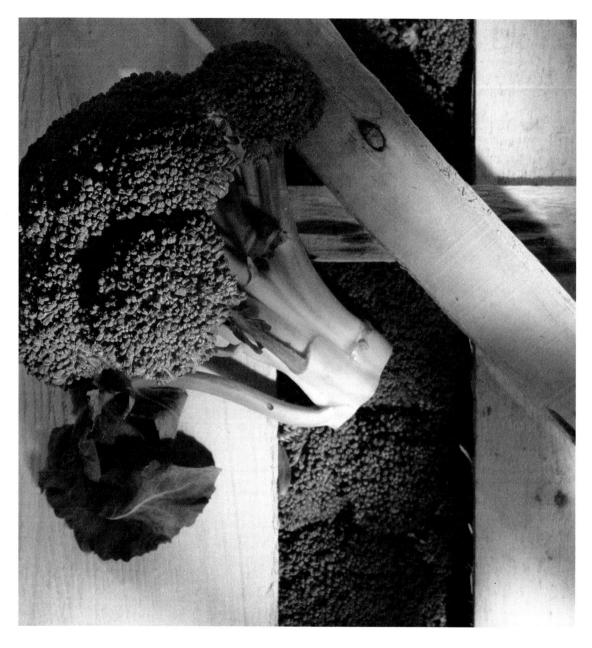

Broccoli leaves and tops are a wonderful source of folic acid and beta-carotene, which the body converts into vitamin A. Broccoli is rich in vitamins B, C, and E, calcium, and iron.

A 110g (4oz) helping of broccoli supplies a third of the calcium, a seventh of the iron, and probably all the vitamin C your body requires in a day.

cervix and bladder); selenium (which protects against cancer of the breast and bowel); zinc (which reduces the risk of cancer of the prostate and boosts immunity); raw fruits and vegetables (which contain anti-oxidant vitamins A, C, and E, and other anti-cancer nutrients) and pulses (which contain anti-cancer agents).

Some specialists believe that you can reduce the risk of cancer by eating live, fermented foods and drinks such as fermented grains, nuts, seeds, and juices, and yoghurt. These encourage the presence of healthy bacteria in the bowel. Other popular foods for preventing cancer are sprouted seeds (including grains).

Excessive alcohol consumption has been correlated with an increased risk of cancer of the mouth, tongue, throat, oesophagus, and liver (especially in smokers). Avoid damaged, stale, diseased, or wilted foods as they are more likely to contain carcinogens. Choose cold-pressed vegetable oils as heat-processed oils may be more likely to contain carcinogens. (Cold-pressed oils are usually darker and more opaque, and some contain sediment). Keep fried foods to a minimum because heating fats (including oils) increases carcinogens and decreases essential fatty acids. Avoid burning or smoking food, and don't eat or drink things too hot.

If you have cancer, it makes good sense to eat nutritious foods and to avoid "empty" calories to help your immune system fight the cancer. If you are taking drugs, a good diet (*the basic healthy diet*) helps you recover faster from their side-effects. Some people have benefited from a *semi-fast diet* for a day or two, followed by a day on raw fruit and vegetables, then a return to *the basic healthy diet*, but with animal protein replaced by vegetable protein (grains, pulses, etc.). A *semi-fast diet* one day a week thereafter may be helpful. Some experts recommend a diet containing a large proportion of raw fruit and vegetables (especially carrots, apples, beetroot, cabbage, broccoli, and cauliflower). You should cut out dairy foods (except for fresh, untreated milk – but check that it has been tested for TB and brucellosis), meat, and fish out of this diet completely, and reduce fats to 10-20 per cent of your total calorie intake. (See **The basic healthy diet** pp. 12-13, **Foods, nutrients, and ailments** pp. 80-2, **The semi-fast diet** p. 90.)

▲ Fibre; raw fruit and vegetables; fermented foods (including yoghurt); sprouted seeds; vitamins A, B6, C, and E; selenium, zinc.
▼ Saturated fat; excessive alcohol; "empty" calories; salt-cured, salt-pickled, smoked, diseased, stale, fried, or burned foods.

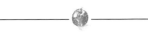

Candidiasis (yeast infection)

Candidiasis is believed to result from an overgrowth of the yeast-like fungus *Candida albicans* in the bowel. It may be associated with thrush in the mouth, vagina, nappy (diaper) area, or nails. The healthy bowel contains 1.4-2.3kg (3-5lb) of micro-organisms, some of which are yeasts. These micro-organisms help with digestion, contribute to the bulk of the bowel motions, mop up potentially dangerous substances, and produce nutrients, such as vitamin K. Sometimes the balance of micro-organisms is disturbed; *Candida* can then multiply and take over the bowel. Overgrowth is most likely if you are diabetic, produce little gastric acid, eat a diet based on meat, sugar, and starch, with little fibre, or have taken certain kinds of antibiotics.

Your diet can stimulate the growth of *Candida*. If you eat a lot of refined carbohydrates, and drink too much alcohol, you feed the organisms with what they need to multiply. If you are sensitive to one or more foods (see *Food sensitivity*) you could have a predisposition to candidiasis. If your diet is poor you could be lacking iron, zinc, magnesium, vitamins A, C, and E, and flavonoids. This could make you less resistant to infection. If you have untreated or out-of-control *diabetes* you increase your risk of *Candida* overgrowth because of the raised levels of sugar throughout your body. If you eat a lot of yeast-containing foods (see p.92) you could increase the risk of *Candida* overgrowth by altering the balance of organisms in the bowel.

Candidiasis is thought to lead to symptoms arising from many parts of the body besides the bowel partly because it may trigger *food sensitivity*. Your symptoms may be worse after eating refined carbohydrates or yeast-containing foods. A dietary change is helpful for symptoms arising from *Candida* overgrowth in the bowel. It helps reduce the overgrowth and sometimes gets rid of it completely; it aids the action of anti-*Candida* drugs, and it prevents recurrences. The diet you need is relatively limited, so choose foods wisely. You may feel "flu-like" for about three weeks after beginning the diet.

Diet Changing your diet helps in five ways. First your diet can starve the organisms. Cut out added sugar, other refined carbohydrates, alcohol, and foods containing large amounts of natural sugar, such as milk, fruit, and fruit juice. Do not drink more than two or three cups of coffee or tea a day because caffeine stimulates

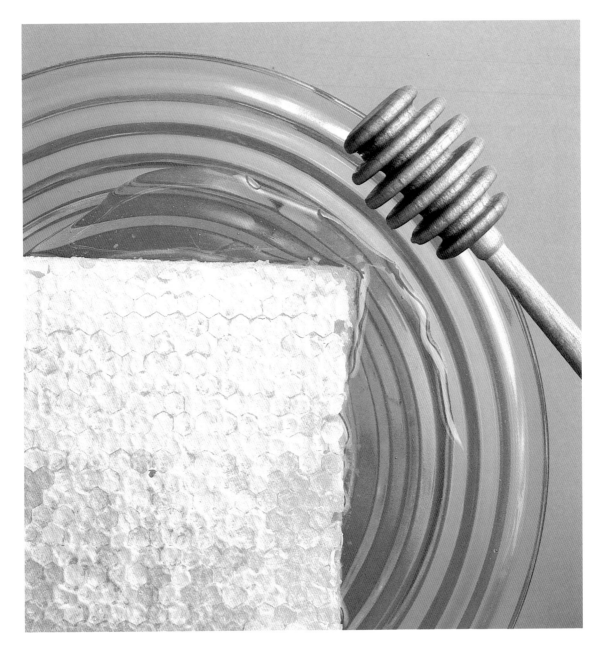

Honey's exact chemical content is unknown, but it is 75% sugar (fructose or fruit sugar, plus sucrose) and 20% water. It also contains minerals (iron, copper, manganese, calcium, magnesium, and phosphorus), vitamins (thiamine, riboflavin, niacin, pantothenic acid, B6, biotin, folic acid, and C), flower flavourings, pollens, enzymes, and antibiotics.

insulin production. This initially releases sugar, which favours *Candida* growth. Reduce total carbohydrates to 60-80gm (2-3oz) per day. Second, your diet can kill *Candida*. Eat two crushed cloves of raw garlic three times a day. Step up your intake of foods containing vitamin B (particularly biotin and vitamins B6 and B12). Fresh, raw, leafy green vegetables and oils containing monounsaturated fatty acids (like olive oil) also act as anti-*Candida* agents. Third, your diet can replace the overgrowth of *Candida* with "healthier" micro-organisms. Eat unpasteurized, live yoghurt two or three times a day. The lactobacilli colonize the bowel as the *Candida* die off, and also produce biotin. Fourth, you can avoid adding fungi to the bowel by rejecting foods containing yeasts, moulds, and other fungi. Fifth, your diet can boost your immune system. Check you are eating enough iron, zinc, magnesium, vitamins A, C, and E, and flavonoids.

Ideally, begin with a two-day *semi-fast diet* (but avoid fruit juices). The next day, eat only raw vegetables or vegetable juices. Continue with the dietary changes outlined above for as long as it takes to clear your symptoms. When you are better, gradually introduce other foods. Prevent recurrences by eating *the basic healthy diet*. (See **The basic healthy diet** pp. 12-13, **Foods, nutrients, and ailments** pp. 80-2, **The semi-fast diet** p. 90.)

▲ Raw garlic; vitamin B; fresh, raw, green leafy vegetables; olive oil; unpasteurized (live) yoghurt.

▼ Refined carbohydrates (especially added sugar); alcohol; milk; fruit; fruit juice; total carbohydrate; yeast (or other mould-containing foods); excessive coffee and tea.

Cataracts

A cataract is a disturbance in the structure of the eye's lens that distorts or blocks light rays. The lens is nourished by the fluid around it, and a deficiency of nutrients in this fluid may cause damage. This can result from a poor diet and/or a reduced blood supply. The sort of diet (high in total and saturated fats) that contributes to degenerative conditions such as *arterial disease* and *arthritis* can also cause cataracts. The high blood sugar of *diabetes* can lead to cataracts, too, since sugar from the lens fluid is concentrated in the lens. Sugar derivatives then alter the crystalline structure of the lens to cause a cataract. Excess added sugar in the diet can also form cataracts even without *diabetes*.

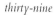

Diet You can help prevent cataracts by eating enough vitamins A, C, and E, manganese, selenium, and zinc. To stop cataracts worsening, cut down animal protein and saturated fat. Avoid added sugar, and eat spinach and raw vegetables. (See **The basic healthy diet** pp. 12-13, **Foods, nutrients, and ailments** pp. 80-2.)

▲ Vitamins A, C, E; manganese, selenium, zinc; spinach; raw vegetables.

▼ Animal protein; saturated fat; added sugar.

Catarrh (mucus)

Diet Avoid refined carbohydrates, fried foods, and caffeine. Cut down dairy foods, animal protein, and alcohol. Eat plenty of raw fruits and vegetables, and enough vitamins A, B, C and flavonoids. Onions, garlic, and yarrow, juniper berry or elderflower teas may help. If you suspect *food sensitivity* pinpoint "culprit" foods. (See **The basic healthy diet** pp. 12-13, **Foods, nutrients, and ailments** pp. 80-2, **The exclusion diet** pp. 91-3.)

▲ Raw fruit and vegetables; vitamins A, B, C, and flavonoids; onion and garlic; yarrow, juniper berry, or elderflower teas.

▼ Refined carbohydrates; fried foods; tea, coffee, cocoa, and cola; dairy foods; animal protein; alcohol.

Circulation problems

Your diet can improve or prevent chilblains, cold extremities, and Raynaud's phenomenon. Poor circulation can be caused by a diet that makes the blood too sticky. Hardening of the arteries and atheroma also slow circulation. If your diet is high in refined carbohydrates you are unlikely to be receiving optimum levels of nutrients. This can lead to a chemical imbalance in the fluid bathing the body's cells, which prevents the blood flowing freely.

Diet Eat *the basic healthy diet* and take dietary measures for *arterial disease* and abnormal blood stickiness (see p.29), if necessary. Chilblains may respond to a diet rich in vitamin E and flavonoids. Avoid alcohol, and add spices to food or drinks. Helpful herbal teas include yarrow, elderflower, rosemary, feverfew, peppermint, and chamomile flower. (See **The basic healthy diet** pp. 12-13, **Foods, nutrients, and ailments** pp. 80-2.)

▲ Vitamin E and flavonoids; cayenne, ginger, mustard, horseradish, and cinnamon; yarrow, elderflower, rosemary, feverfew, peppermint, or chamomile flower teas.

Colic

Dietary causes include *wind* (gas), *constipation*, overeating, poor chewing, hunger, a poor diet, too much caffeine, *food sensitivity*, certain foods, such as green apples, and *lead poisoning*.

Diet   Avoid overeating, and drinking with meals. If you suspect a *food sensitivity*, pinpoint your "culprit" foods. Try eating foods rich in zinc, calcium, magnesium, potassium, and vitamins B, D, and E, and avoiding caffeine. Peppermint or ginger tea may help. Some breast-fed babies are sensitive to foods in breast milk, or they may get colic from anxiety-provoked substances in the milk. It may help to space out your calorie intake and eat between feeds. (See **The basic healthy diet** pp. 12-13, **Foods, nutrients, and ailments** pp. 80-2, **The exclusion diet** pp. 91-3.)

▲ Vitamins B, D, and E; zinc, calcium, magnesium, potassium; peppermint or ginger tea.

▼ "Culprit" foods; coffee, tea, cocoa, cola.

Confusion

Some causes of confusion have a dietary link. *Arterial disease* and *high blood pressure*, for instance, can reduce the circulation of blood in the brain, and can eventually cause confusion.

Diet   Take steps to arrest *arterial disease* and *high blood pressure* (if necessary). Avoid *low blood sugar*. Identify "culprit" foods. Eat more raw fruit and vegetables. Increase foods rich in calcium, magnesium, zinc, lecithin and essential fatty acids, and vitamins B, C, and E. Aluminium is still under suspicion, so get rid of aluminium cookware, and filter water high in aluminium. Avoid salt and white flour. (See **The basic healthy diet** pp. 12-13, **Foods, nutrients, and ailments** pp. 80-2, **The exclusion diet** pp. 91-3.)

▲ Raw fruit and vegetables; vitamins B, C, and E; calcium, magnesium, zinc, lecithin, essential fatty acids.

▼ "Culprit" foods; white flour; table salt.

Constipation

This is common with a high consumption of refined carbohydrates, and it is responsible for many disorders, including piles, *varicose veins*, and anal fissures. Straining can contribute to a hernia. Prevent constipation by eating *the basic healthy diet*. If you are already a sufferer, eat more foods containing fibre and drink more water.

Diet Eat wholegrain bread and use wholegrain flours. Eat more oats, fruit and vegetables, and drink plenty. (See **The basic healthy diet** pp. 12-13, **Foods, nutrients, and ailments** pp. 80-2.)

▲ Water; wholegrain bread and flour; oats; fruit and vegetables.

▼ Refined carbohydrates.

Cot (crib) death (sudden infant death syndrome)

One in 1421 babies dies suddenly and unexpectedly in the UK, and at post-mortem examination pathologists are unable to find any apparent cause. Research highlights the multifactorial nature of the condition. Diet may have a part to play in some of the deaths. Some babies cannot cope with long intervals between feeds – most cot/crib deaths occur between midnight and mid-day; certainly a few use up their sugar stores and are then unable to use fat stores for energy. Deficiencies of biotin, vitamin E, manganese, or selenium may exist. Many babies have symptoms of minor infection, and many have abnormal fluid in their lung linings.

Diet Try not to leave a gap between feeds longer than three or four hours in very young babies, and not more than six hours in older babies, particularly under six months. If bottle feeding, follow the instructions and never add extra milk powder. If breast feeding, eat a healthy breast-feeding diet (see p. 14) to help combat infection. Lay your baby on the back to sleep. (See **The basic healthy diet** pp. 12-13, **Foods, nutrients, and ailments** pp. 80-2.)

Cramps

A diet that predisposes one to *arterial disease*, poor circulation, *arthritis*, and *rheumatism* can cause cramps, as can *alcoholism*, specific nutritional deficiencies, and excessive sweating.

Diet Cramps may respond to a diet rich in zinc, calcium, magnesium, and potassium. Vitamin-D-rich foods enable calcium to be used properly, and vitamin-E-rich foods facilitate sugar release in muscles. Some people find more vitamins B and C and flavonoids, cloves, cider vinegar, ginger, and peppermint tea helpful. Too much *and* too little salt can cause cramps. (See **The basic healthy diet** pp. 12-13, **Foods, nutrients, and ailments** pp. 80-2.)

▲ Vitamins B, C, D, and E; flavonoids; zinc, calcium, magnesium, potassium; cloves; cider vinegar and ginger; peppermint tea; salt.

▼ Salt (if necessary).

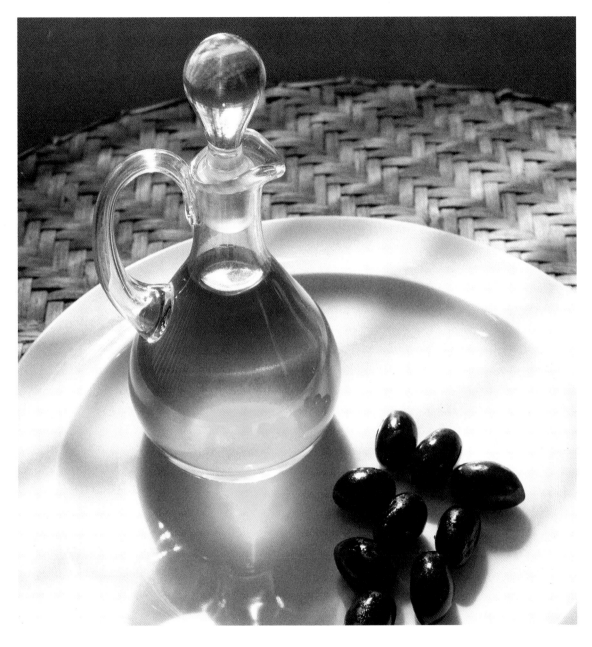

Olive oil has an attractive and distinctive scent, especially the green-gold first pressing of freshly picked olives. This is the most precious of the various grades of oil and should be kept in a cool, dark place, and refrigerated only in hot weather. Olive oil contains a high proportion of mono-unsaturated fatty acids, which help keep the heart and arteries healthy.

Depression

Depression can be associated with low levels of vitamins B and C, calcium, iron, magnesium, potassium, and zinc; *candidiasis*; excess caffeine consumption (more than eight strong cups of coffee a day); *low blood sugar, food sensitivity*, and insufficient gastric acid.

Many depressed people crave carbohydrates. This is common in people suffering from *obesity*, post-natal (post-partum) depression, the *pre-menstrual syndrome*, and seasonal affective disorder. This depression and craving may reflect low levels of the neurotransmitter serotonin in the brain. Increase your serotonin levels by eating more low-protein tryptophan-rich complex carbohydrate snacks (see p. 56). Vitamin B6 is necessary for serotonin production, which may explain why the contraceptive pill, which lowers B6 levels, can cause depression. Other people get depressed because they have low levels of noradrenaline in their brain. Tyrosine and phenylalanine raise noradrenaline levels and they do this best if you eat meals high in protein and low in carbohydrates.

Diet Experiment to find out whether your depression is relieved by high-carbohydrate, low-protein meals, or the reverse. Avoid *low blood sugar* and eat more foods rich in flavonoids. Reduce your caffeine consumption. If you suspect a *food sensitivity*, pinpoint your "culprit" foods. Try eating proteins and starches separately. Borage, chamomile flower, chervil, lavender flower, and peppermint teas may help. Cloves, cayenne and mangoes can be beneficial. (See **The basic healthy diet** pp. 12-13, **Foods, nutrients, and ailments** pp. 80-2, **The exclusion diet** pp. 91-3.)

▲ Carbohydrates or protein; vitamins B, C, and flavonoids; calcium, iron, magnesium, potassium, zinc; borage, chamomile flower, chervil, lavender flower, and peppermint teas.

▼ Carbohydrates or protein (whichever necessary); coffee, tea, cocoa, cola; "culprit" foods.

Diabetes

Altering your diet can prevent maturity-onset diabetes and if you are insulin-dependent can reduce the amount of insulin needed – but consult your doctor before making dietary changes.

Diet Lose excess weight and stop eating refined carbohydrates. Coarsely ground wholegrains give more protection than finely ground wholegrains. Eat more raw vegetables and fruits (especially carrots, onions, and green leafy vegetables), whole oats, lentils,

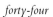

peas, and beans. Make sure you eat enough foods rich in vitamins A, B, C, E, and flavonoids, chromium, magnesium, manganese, potassium, vanadium, zinc, and essential fatty acids. Decrease the amount of animal protein and saturated fat in your diet. Eat less salt, reduce caffeine-containing drinks, and cut alcohol down or out. (See **The basic healthy diet** pp. 12-13, **Foods, nutrients, and ailments** pp. 80-2. **The weight-reducing diet** pp. 87-9.)

▲ Unrefined carbohydrates; whole oats; pulses (beans and peas); lentils; raw vegetables and fruits; vitamins A, B, C, E, and flavonoids; chromium, magnesium, manganese, potassium, vanadium, zinc, essential fatty acids.

▼ Refined carbohydrates (including added sugar); animal protein; saturated fats; salt; alcohol; tea, coffee, cocoa, cola.

Diverticular disease

Researchers believe that diverticular disease is caused by years of eating a diet low in fibre and high in refined carbohydrates.

Diet Eating *the basic healthy diet* with extra fibre-rich foods. Cut refined carbohydrates down or out. (See **The basic healthy diet** pp. 12-13, **Foods, nutrients, and ailments** pp. 80-2.)

▲ Unrefined carbohydrates; raw and cooked vegetables and fruit; pulses, oats, nuts, seeds.

▼ Refined carbohydrates (including added sugar).

Ear problems

Repeated middle ear infection may respond to dietary measures for *infection* and *catarrh*. Breastfed babies have fewer middle ear infections. Menière's disease may be associated with a relative niacin deficiency or a *low blood sugar* tendency. Aluminium toxicity may be linked with otosclerosis. A long-term protein deficiency or premature *ageing* can lead to deafness.

Diet For ear infections eat a diet to counteract *infection* and *catarrh*. For Menière's disease eat more niacin, and avoid *low blood sugar* swings. For otosclerosis eat more vitamins A and D, and calcium, and enough protein. Avoid aluminium cookware, salt, and white flour and filter drinking water. (See **The basic healthy diet** pp. 12-13, **Foods, nutrients, and ailments** pp. 80-2.)

▲ (For Menière's disease) niacin. (For otosclerosis) vitamins A, D; calcium.

▲ (For otosclerosis) aluminium.

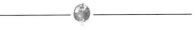

Eyes, dryness of

Dryness of the eyes occurs when you have too little tear fluid and it is associated with a roughening of the cornea. Adequate amounts of essential fatty acids in *the basic healthy diet* help prevent this condition. A shortage of vitamin A is a common cause.

Diet   Eat more foods rich in essential fatty acids and vitamin A (from vegetable and animal sources). Researchers have discovered that vitamin A from food is more effective than vitamin A supplements in treating severe eye problems. (See **The basic healthy diet** pp. 12-13, **Foods, nutrients, and ailments** pp. 80-2.) ▲ Essential fatty acids; vitamin A.

Food sensitivity

Food sensitivity can cause asthma, eczema, migraine, arthritis, *depression*, *behaviour and learning problems*, diarrhoea, *gallstones*, *tiredness*, fluid retention, weight fluctuation, food craving, obesity, *catarrh*, epilepsy, *mouth ulcers*, recurrent abdominal pain, Crohn's disease, skin roughness, and urticaria. Sometimes it is easy to relate the symptom to a particular food, but often the link is not obvious; you may be sensitive to many foods and to the very foods you crave most. Pinning down a "culprit" food can be difficult if it is one you eat all the time, or if your symptoms are vague or longstanding.

One difficulty with tracking down a "culprit" food is that symptoms may appear within seconds, minutes, hours, or days. Food sensitivity may be triggered by one of the first foods given as a baby. There may be vague symptoms after eating the food (such as flushing, red ears, diarrhoea, irritability, or stomach ache), but these tend to subside. However, days, months, or even years later, that same food can trigger symptoms once more. A poor diet, lack of sleep, infection, distress, digestive problems, extremes of temperature, a smoky or polluted atmosphere, certain medicinal drugs, and pollutants in food may together weaken your immune system and cause it to react unusually to a normally innocuous food. Food sensitivity may occur after *gastroenteritis*, antibiotic drugs, malnutrition, or jaundice.

In coeliac disease the bowel cannot absorb gluten. This commonly starts in infancy and can also follow *gastroenteritis*.

The commonest "culprits" with asthma are manufactured "fruit" and fizzy drinks, nuts, sodium benzoate, milk, eggs, wheat, cheese, yeast, fish, and fried food.

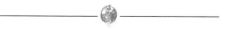

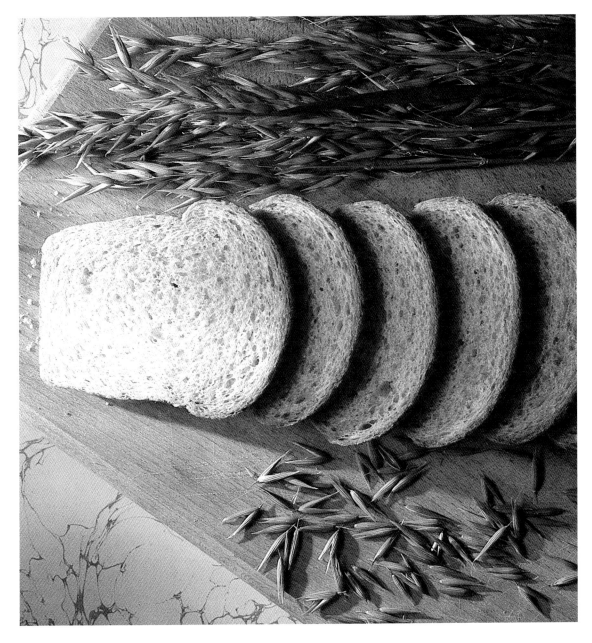

Wholegrains *have more protein, fat, iron, thiamine, riboflavin, and niacin than the refined grains used to make white bread and flour. They also contain large amounts of valuable cereal fibre. Choose wholegrains or foods made with the whole of the grain (such as wholewheat flour), because of the many nutrients in the bran and wheatgerm.*

Possible "culprits" with migraine include oranges, chocolate, sugar, cheese, alcohol (especially red wine), wheat, eggs, coffee, tea, cola, milk, beef, corn, yeast, pickled fish, cured meat, bananas, broad beans, sausages, sauerkraut, and liver. One in ten migraine sufferers is food-sensitive. Try cutting out caffeine, alcohol and added sugar first. If you have migraine your blood may be abnormally "sticky" (see p. 29). Other potential "culprits" are foods containing salicylates (see p. 92). Citric acid, found in cola and citrus fruit, can cause *depression*, *confusion*, hyperactivity, *anxiety*, clumsiness, and *tiredness*. It has also been linked with *schizophrenia*.

Diet Identify "culprit" foods with an exclusion diet. You may not have to avoid these foods forever, though coeliac sufferers need professional advice. Sometimes, after avoiding the food for several months, it is possible to reintroduce it gradually, though you may only be able to eat it every few days. Your symptoms may worsen after stopping the food, but continued avoidance brings relief.

Ideally breastfeed completely for at least six months, especially if there is a family history of allergy. Avoid large amounts of any one food when pregnant or breastfeeding. Delay giving your baby wheat until eight months; citrus fruits and juices until nine months; fish ten months; cows' milk eleven months; eggs one year; and nuts, fruit, and vegetables with pips or seeds even longer.

Lower your risk of food sensitivity by avoiding refined and processed foods. More essential fatty acids may help, and extra foods rich in vitamins A and C may be useful as well.

Some food-sensitive people produce insufficient gastric acid. This can lead to poor absorption of nutrients such as calcium and iron and it may help to eat meat at different times from carbohydrates; have some vinegar with meat, fish and eggs, and eat more foods containing niacin.

If you have been eating poorly, you may be short of iron, magnesium, zinc, and vitamin B, so eat more foods rich in these nutrients until you are better. Cutting down on alcohol may help. Foods rich in vitamin B6 may make asthma less likely, and foods rich in selenium may improve eczema (watercress may help, too).

Foods rich in vitamins B6, C, and E, and garlic and ginger may help migraine. These, along with essential fatty acids, reduce the stickiness of the blood. Feverfew leaves relieve some migraine headaches (but do not eat feverfew for more than 14 consecutive days). (See **The basic healthy diet** pp. 12-13, **Foods, nutrients, and ailments** pp. 80-2, **The exclusion diet** pp. 91-3.)

▲ Essential fatty acids; vitamins A, B, C; iron, magnesium, selenium, zinc. (For asthma) hyssop, thyme, chamomile flower teas. (For eczema) selenium; watercress. (For migraine) vitamins E; garlic, ginger, feverfew, oily fish; rosemary and lavender flower teas.

▼ "Culprit" foods; alcohol; highly refined or processed food.

Gallstones

Vegetarians are less likely to have gallstones and people who are 20 per cent overweight are twice as likely to develop them. *Food sensitivity* is responsible for many symptoms – the most likely "culprit" foods are eggs, pork, and onions. Constipation encourages gallstones too.

Diet   Always eat breakfast. Reduce your intake of saturated fats, animal protein and refined carbohydrates; eat more foods containing lecithin and essential fatty acids, vitamins C and E, zinc, and fibre. Foods containing salicylates (see p.92) may help prevent gallstones. Raw dandelion leaves, horseradish and artichoke are helpful, as are dandelion, chamomile flower, and parsley teas. (See **The basic healthy diet** pp. 12-13, **Foods, nutrients, and ailments** pp. 80-2, **The weight-reducing diet** pp. 87-9, **The exclusion diet** pp. 91-3.)

▲ Fibre; lecithin and essential fatty acids; vitamins C and E; zinc; dandelion leaves, horse radish and artichoke; dandelion, chamomile flower, and parsley teas.

▼ Saturated fats; animal protein; refined carbohydrates (including added sugar); "culprit" foods.

Gastroenteritis and food poisoning

The micro-organisms that cause gastroenteritis enter the digestive tract via infected food or hands. The infection spreads easily, and if you have gastroenteritis it is best not to handle or prepare food; but if you must, wash your hands well first. To prevent traveller's diarrhoea, wash your hands before eating; drink bottled, purified, or boiled water, avoid ice, peel fruit or rinse it in bottled water, and avoid salads washed in tap water.

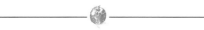

Food poisoning is caused by bacterial toxins in infected food. Thorough cooking destroys the bacteria, but not the toxins. Raw seafood can be a source of infection. It is important to: buy eggs that originate from a salmonella-tested flock; avoid soft cheese during pregnancy and at other times to buy it from a store with a high turnover; avoid buying dented cans or time-expired food; avoid storing cooked and uncooked meat together; cook raw food thoroughly; reheat leftovers thoroughly; allow enough time for defrosting; follow instructions precisely for microwave ovens and cook-chill packages; and keep surfaces and utensils clean.

Breastfeeding protects babies to some extent. Young children can readily become dangerously dehydrated as a result of gastroenteritis. Get professional help for vomiting lasting over an hour in a baby, or more than four hours in an older child or adult, or which is severe or violent; or for diarrhoea lasting longer than a day.

Diet Drink plenty of liquids to replace lost fluid, but avoid alcohol. If you are vomiting take frequent sips of water. You lose a lot of potassium with diarrhoea, so eat potassium-rich foods. Raw garlic helps combat infection. Live yoghurt may help rebalance bowel bacteria. (See **Foods, nutrients, and ailments** pp. 80-2.)

▲ Fluid; potassium.

▼ Alcohol.

Goitre

Iodine is necessary for the production of the hormone thyroxine in the thyroid gland, as is vitamin C. Iodine deficiency, found in areas with insufficient iodine in the soil, can lead to goitre. Goitre-inducing chemicals occur in vegetables of the brassica family (e.g. cabbage), but if there is enough iodine in the soil, these chemicals do not usually cause goitre. Moreover, cooking reduces the level by up to a half. A goitre can indicate an over- or underactive thyroid. Both conditions can be associated with insufficient gastric acid so eat more niacin, take vinegar with meat, fish and eggs, and eat protein and carbohydrate separately.

Diet In an iodine-deficient area eat more foods rich in iodine and vitamin C. An unexplained goitre may be helped by avoiding brassica vegetables. (See **The basic healthy diet** pp. 12-13, **Foods, nutrients, and ailments** pp. 80-2.)

▲ Iodine (if necessary); niacin and vitamin C.

▼ Brassica vegetables (if necessary).

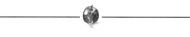

Gout

Gout is a form of arthritis in which uric acid crystals are deposited in the joints. Vegetarians have less gout and if you are more than 5 per cent overweight, you have an increased chance of developing it.

Diet Gout is made worse by purine-containing foods (red meat, game, offal/organ meats, fish, fish roes, shellfish, wholegrains, asparagus, cauliflower, mushrooms, spinach, and pulses/beans and peas), meat stock, alcohol (especially beer), excess fruit (the fructose increases urate production), yeast-based flavourings, *lead poisoning*, refined carbohydrates and saturated fats. Lose excess weight, drink more fluid, and eat more high-fibre foods, green leafy vegetables (their folic acid reduces uric acid levels), celery, parsley, and watercress, and foods rich in zinc, magnesium, and vitamin C (which increases the loss of uric acid in the urine). Feverfew leaves reduce the inflammation and pain, but avoid eating these for more than 14 consecutive days. Raw vegetable juices help, as do dandelion, nettle, and meadowsweet teas. (See **The basic healthy diet** pp. 12-13, **Foods, nutrients, and ailments** pp. 80-2, **The weight-reducing diet** pp. 87-9.)

▲ Fibre; fluid; green leafy vegetables; celery, parsley, and watercress; vitamin C; magnesium, zinc; feverfew; raw vegetable juices; dandelion root or leaf, nettle, and meadowsweet teas.

▼ Purine-containing foods; alcohol (especially beer); excess fruit; yeast-based flavourings; vinegar; refined carbohydrates (including added sugar); saturated fats.

Gum disease

If your gums are soft and bleed often you may need more vitamin C. If your diet is poor you are more likely to get gingivitis, and if you eat a diet high in refined carbohydrates you are likely to develop a thick film of plaque over your teeth. Unless removed this soon forms tartar, which increases the risk of gum disease.

Diet Reduce your intake of refined carbohydrates (including added sugar). Eat plenty of high-fibre foods, including green leafy vegetables, and make sure you eat enough foods containing vitamins A and C, and flavonoids. (See **The basic healthy diet** pp. 12-13, **Foods, nutrients, and ailments** pp. 80-2.)

▲ Fibre; vitamins A and C, and flavonoids; green leafy vegetables.

▼ Refined carbohydrates (including added sugar).

Hair loss

Hair loss may occur generally all over the scalp; selectively, as in male pattern baldness; or in patches. If you are deficient in protein, zinc, vitamins B and C; if you have *anaemia*, or *diabetes*; or if you have been on a diet, you may have hair loss. It is thought that male pattern loss is increased by the typical refined westernized diet. This may eventually lead to reduced circulation in the scalp, with consequent hair thinning in those hereditarily susceptible. Alopecia areata can be associated with *food sensitivity*.

Diet   Eat enough foods rich in protein, iron, zinc, and vitamins B and C. Identify "culprit" foods if you have alopecia areata. Cut down meat, saturated fat, and refined carbohydrates, and eat more fruit and vegetables. (See **The basic healthy diet** pp. 12-13, **Foods, nutrients, and ailments** p. 80-2, **The exclusion diet** pp. 91-3.)

▲ Fruit and vegetables; unsaturated fats; vitamins B and C; protein; iron, zinc.

▼ "Culprit" foods; meat; saturated fats; refined carbohydrates.

Headache

Headaches can result from the nitrites in cured meats, monosodium glutamate, potassium deficiency from a poor diet or diarrhoea, dehydration, *high blood pressure*, a hangover, *low blood sugar*, aluminium poisoning, *candidiasis*, *food sensitivity*, too much coffee, and *lead poisoning*. Migraines are sometimes linked to *food sensitivity*. More than four cups of strong coffee a day can cause a headache, but if you are used to caffeine-containing drinks and then go without, you may suffer a withdrawal headache.

Diet Limit caffeine-containing drinks and eat more foods rich in calcium and magnesium, and more oily fish. Identify "culprit" foods if you suspect a *food sensitivity*, and eat foods rich in potassium if you have diarrhoea. Avoid aluminium poisoning (see p. 41). Alter your diet if you suffer from *high blood pressure*, *low blood sugar* swings, or *candidiasis*. Feverfew (do not eat this for more than 14 consecutive days), mint, rosemary, ginger root, chamomile flower, lavender flower, limeflower teas may be useful. (See **The basic healthy diet** pp. 12-13, **Foods, nutrients, and ailments** pp. 80-2, **The exclusion diet** pp. 91-3.)

▲ Calcium, magnesium; oily fish; feverfew leaves; mint, rosemary, ginger root, chamomile flower, lavender flower, limeflower teas.

▼ Caffeine; "culprit" foods.

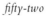

High blood pressure

High blood pressure increases the risk of a stroke, kidney disease, and a heart attack. You may be able to reduce high blood pressure by changing your diet and losing excess weight. You should restrict salt, but increase the amount of potassium in your diet. Deficiencies of calcium or magnesium may be associated with high blood pressure, as may *lead poisoning*. Vegetarians have lower blood pressure than meat-eaters. People who drink alcohol moderately have lower blood pressure than either teetotalers or heavy drinkers. Caffeine-containing drinks cause a temporary rise in blood pressure.

Diet Lose excess weight. Eat more oily fish and more foods rich in potassium, calcium, magnesium, vitamins B, C, D, and E, flavonoids, essential fatty acids and lecithin, fibre, and more raw vegetables, including onions and garlic. Eat less saturated fat. Reduce your intake of salt and added sugar, and drink only small to moderate amounts of alcohol. Some people find a *semi-fast diet* one day a week helps. (See **The basic healthy diet** pp. 12-13, **Foods, nutrients, and ailments** pp. 80-2, **The weight-reducing diet** pp. 87-9, **The semi-fast diet** p. 90.)

▲ Fibre; lecithin; essential fatty acids; oily fish, raw fruit and vegetables (especially onions and garlic); vitamins B, C, D, and E and flavonoids; potassium, calcium, magnesium.

▼ Salt; added sugar; saturated fat; alcohol (if necessary).

Impotence

Impotence is the inability to obtain an erection at all, or for long enough to have satisfactory intercourse. In younger men dietary factors usually take second place to psychosexual and other causes. Prostate problems and *arterial disease* may be responsible, and *low blood sugar* can cause temporary impotence. A diet deficient in iodine, manganese, selenium, or zinc has been linked with some cases, while research has found reducing saturated fats beneficial.

Diet Make sure you are eating *the basic healthy diet*, which contains enough foods rich in iodine, manganese, selenium, and zinc. Avoid *low blood sugar*-induced impotence by eating a high-fibre, low-refined carbohydrate diet. (See **The basic healthy diet** pp. 12-13, **Foods, nutrients, and ailments** pp. 80-2.)

▲ Iodine, manganese, selenium, and zinc (if necessary); fibre.

▼ Saturated fat; refined carbohydrates.

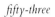

Indigestion

Gastritis can be associated with too much or too little gastric acid – alcohol, milk, caffeine, and fatty or spicy foods can increase acid production. *Food sensitivity* may be a problem. Indigestion often improves with a diet low in refined carbohydrates. Foods rich in vitamin C and zinc may speed up the healing of the stomach lining. Other causes include gallstones, hiatus hernia and *candidiasis*.

Diet Cut down alcohol, milk, caffeine-containing drinks, and fatty foods. If you suspect *food sensitivity* pinpoint your "culprit" foods. Try eating proteins separately from carbohydrates and adding vinegar to meat, fish and eggs, and eat foods rich in vitamins B and C and zinc. Keep meals stress-free, chew well, and do not overeat. Paw-paw (papaya), apples, pineapple, raw cabbage, carrots and ginger may help prevent indigestion and parsley, mint, chamomile flower, blackberry leaf, and juniper berry teas may ease the pain. (See **The basic healthy diet** pp. 12-13, **Foods, nutrients, and ailments** pp. 80-2, **The exclusion diet** pp. 91-3.)

▲ Vitamin C; zinc; paw-paw, apples, pineapple, raw cabbage, carrots, ginger and parsley, mint, chamomile flower, blackberry leaf, and juniper berry teas.

▼ Refined carbohydrates (including added sugar); alcohol; milk; coffee, tea, cocoa, cola; fatty and spicy foods; "culprit" foods.

Infection

A poor diet with a shortage of zinc leads to decreased resistance. Added sugar, *lead poisoning*, and excess caffeine depress immunity and alcohol reduces vitamin B and zinc levels.

Diet Eat foods rich in riboflavin, pantothenic acid, vitamins A, B6, C, D, E, folic acid and flavonoids; zinc, iron, magnesium, copper, iodine, and selenium; essential fatty acids and lecithin. Cut down on refined carbohydrates and alcohol. Crushed raw garlic, spicy food, and raw fruit and vegetables daily will help. Echinacea root tea may be beneficial. (See **The basic healthy diet** pp. 12-13, **Foods, nutrients, and ailments** pp. 80-2.)

▲ Essential fatty acids and lecithin; garlic, spices, raw fruit and vegetables; riboflavin, pantothenic acid, vitamins A, B6, C, D, E, folic acid, and flavonoids; zinc, iron, magnesium, copper, iodine, selenium; echinacea root tea.

▼ Refined carbohydrates; alcohol; excess coffee, tea, cocoa, cola.

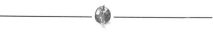

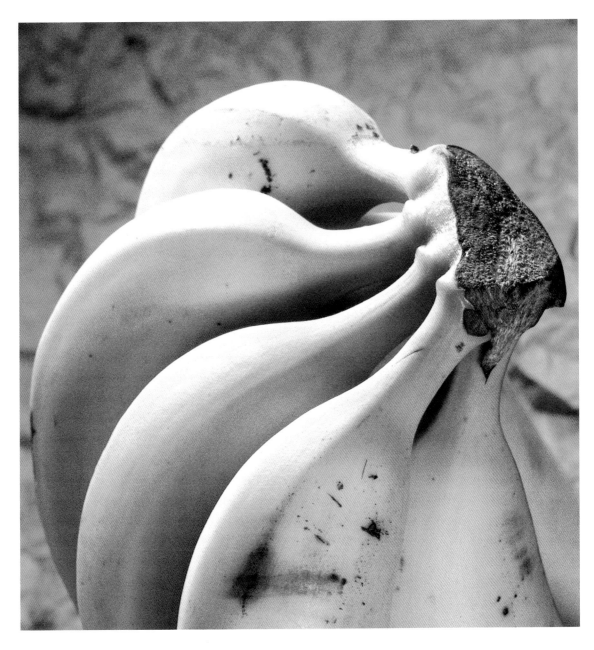

Bananas contain more carbohydrate than most fruits and when they are ripe they are sweet and easily digested. Their high fibre content ensures that the sugars are slowly and smoothly absorbed into the bloodstream, making them a satisfying food. Bananas are also rich in potassium, magnesium, vitamins B6 and C, and the "calming" amino acid tryptophan.

Infertility

There are several dietary reasons for infertility, including severe malnutrition, anorexia nervosa, and repeated, poor-quality weight-loss diets. Gross *obesity* can make a man infertile. Dietary deficiencies of zinc, chromium, manganese, selenium, essential fatty acids, vitamins A, B (especially B6), C, and E and folic acid are associated with infertility. Untreated *food sensitivity* may lead to poor absorption of zinc.

Diet   Lose weight (if necessary). Eat foods rich in zinc, chromium, manganese, selenium, vitamins A, B (especially B6), C, and E, folic acid, and essential fatty acids. Improve your diet at least six months before you wish to start a baby, because dietary changes are slow to enhance fertility. (See **The basic healthy diet** pp. 12-13, **Foods, nutrients, and ailments** pp. 80-2, **The weight-reducing diet** pp. 87-9.)

▲ Essential fatty acids; vitamins A, B, C, and E; folic acid; zinc, chromium, manganese, selenium.

Insomnia

Diet   Eat enough foods rich in calcium, magnesium, manganese, zinc, vitamin B (especially riboflavin, pantothenic acid, B6, and inositol – present in wholegrains, liver, oranges, and nuts), fibre, and essential fatty acids. Raw vegetables, especially onions, garlic, and lettuce, aid sleep. A low-protein source of tryptophan may aid sleep. Dates, bread, bananas, hazelnuts, cauliflower, and potatoes are good sources. Chamomile flower, basil, lemon verbena, lemon balm, and valerian teas may help. In the evening avoid alcohol, caffeine, and nightmare-inducing foods. (See **The basic healthy diet** pp. 12-13, **Foods, nutrients, and ailments** pp. 80-2.)

▲ Fibre; low-protein, tryptophan-containing foods; vitamin B, essential fatty acids; calcium, magnesium, manganese, zinc; raw vegetables (especially onions, garlic, and lettuce); chamomile flower, basil, lemon verbena, lemon balm, and valerian teas.

▼ Alcohol; coffee, tea, cocoa, cola; protein.

Irritable bowel syndrome

This may be caused by jerky, non-rhythmical movement of the muscles in the wall of the colon.

Diet Eat more fruit and vegetables as their fibre counteracts the

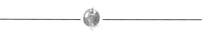

spasm of the bowel. Drink plenty of water and avoid alcohol, tea, and coffee. A few sufferers have *candidiasis* of the bowel instead; others can't drink milk because of lactose (milk sugar) intolerance. *Food sensitivity* is a common problem, so try to identify any "culprit" foods. You may be short of several nutrients because of chronic diarrhoea, so avoid eating "empty" calories. Some people find it helps to eat proteins and starches at separate meals. Try to make mealtimes relaxing occasions. Meadowsweet and chamomile flower teas may be useful. (See **The basic healthy diet** pp. 12-13, **Foods, nutrients, and ailments** pp. 80-2, **The exclusion diet** pp. 91-3.)

▲ Fruit and vegetables; water; meadowsweet and chamomile teas.

▼ Alcohol; tea, coffee, cocoa, cola; refined carbohydrates (especially added sugar); "culprit" foods.

Jet lag

Diet Drink plenty of water-based drinks. Flying often leads to dehydration due to air conditioning and the small size of drinks served. Avoid alcohol because it may dehydrate, and reduce sleep quality. Some people benefit from a *semi-fast* the day they fly.

Kidney stones

Diet Reduce your intake of animal protein, added sugar and alcohol, and eat more fibre. Drink enough water to produce at least 2.5 litres (4.5 pints/2 quarts) of urine daily. For calcium oxalate stones, eat more foods rich in magnesium, potassium and vitamin B6, and eat less saturated fat. Reduce your consumption of oxalic acid by drinking less tea, coffee, and cocoa, and avoiding spinach, rhubarb, sweet potato, cucumber, celery, peanuts, grapefruit, beans, and carrots. For uric acid or cystine stones, eat more alkali-forming foods (see pp.80-2). For uric acid stones, eat less purine-containing food (see p.51). (See **The basic healthy diet** pp. 12-13, **Foods, nutrients, and ailments** pp. 80-2.)

▲ (For all stones) fibre; magnesium and potassium; water. (For calcium oxalate stones) magnesium; vitamin B6. (For uric acid and cystine stones) alkali-forming foods.

▼ (For all stones) animal protein; added sugar; alcohol. (For calcium oxalate stones) tea, coffee, cocoa, spinach, rhubarb, sweet potato, cucumber, celery, peanuts, grapefruit, beans, and carrots. (For uric acid stones) purine-containing foods.

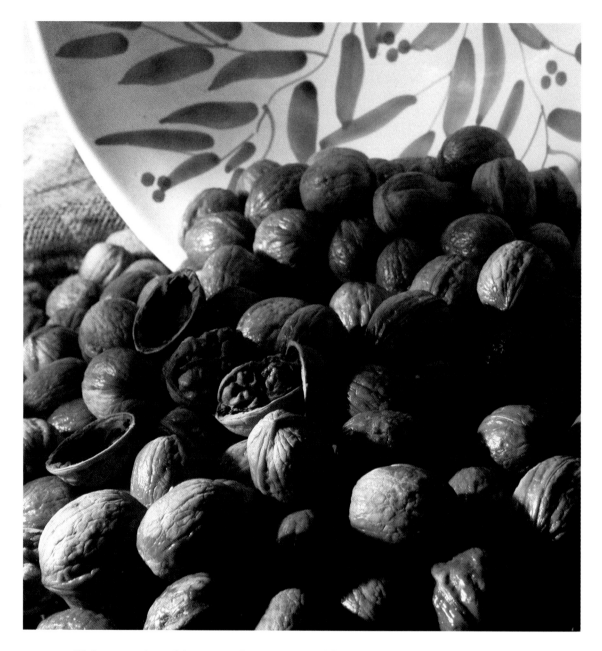

Walnuts *contain useful amounts of protein, fibre, minerals (magnesium, phosphorus, iron, calcium, copper, and zinc), vitamins (A, thiamine, B6, C, E, pantothenic acid, biotin, and folic acid) and essential fatty acids. Their fats are more polyunsaturated than the other dessert nuts, and their cold-pressed oil makes a delicious salad dressing.*

Lead poisoning

Lead poisoning is associated with *behaviour and learning problems*, decreased immunity, *arterial disease*, and *gout*. The major source of lead is food, but water can be an important source. Some foods increase and others decrease the risk of poisoning.

Diet Eat less animal fat and alcohol, and more foods rich in vitamins C, D, and E, calcium, chromium, iron, selenium, zinc, protein, and fibre. Garlic reduces some signs of lead poisoning. Avoid dented cans, since lead sealant can escape into the food. Do not leave food in opened cans. Avoid cooking in earthenware pottery since the glaze may contain lead. (See **The basic healthy diet** pp. 12-13, **Foods, nutrients, and ailments** pp. 80-2.)

▲ Protein; fibre; vitamins C, D, and E; calcium, chromium, iron, selenium, zinc; garlic.

▼ Animal fat; alcohol.

Low blood sugar

A poor diet can cause your blood sugar level to swing outside normal limits. Low blood sugar swings can be associated with *depression, behaviour and learning problems, confusion, tiredness, impotence, insomnia*, migraine, epilepsy, *alcoholism*, and inadequately controlled *diabetes*.

Diet Increase the fibre in your diet as this slows the absorption of sugars and keeps the blood sugar level within normal limits. Too much refined carbohydrate causes the blood sugar level to rise quickly; the pancreas responds by producing a lot of insulin, which can send the blood sugar level abnormally low and make you crave more refined carbohydrate. Fibre from apples; oats and pulses helps keep blood sugar levels normal, and chromium, magnesium, manganese, potassium, selenium, zinc, and vitamin B are useful.

Alcohol makes a low blood sugar more likely. This is important in alcoholics (see *Alcoholism*) because low blood sugar swings make them crave more alcohol. *Food sensitivity* may be responsible for 75 per cent of low blood sugar problems. Caffeine can lead to a low blood sugar. (See **The basic healthy diet** pp. 12-13, **Foods, nutrients, and ailments** pp. 80-2, **The exclusion diet** pp. 91-3.)

▲ Fibre; vitamin B; chromium, magnesium, manganese, potassium, selenium, zinc.

▼ Refined carbohydrates; alcohol; "culprit" foods; coffee, tea, cocoa, and cola.

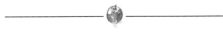

Memory loss

Diet   Eat foods rich in riboflavin, niacin and vitamin B12, iron and magnesium. Memory loss may be associated with the accumulation of the "age pigment" lipofuscin in brain cells. Adequate amounts of vitamin E may slow this process. Too much alcohol impairs the memory. Lecithin provides the building blocks for the production of the neurotransmitter acetyl choline, responsible for storing recent memory. (See **The basic healthy diet** pp. 12-13, **Foods, nutrients, and ailments** pp. 80-2.)

▲ Riboflavin, niacin and vitamins B12, and E; iron, magnesium, manganese, zinc; lecithin.

▼ Alcohol.

Menopausal problems

Diet   Avoid caffeine, which increases calcium loss, and eat enough foods rich in vitamin C plus flavonoids to help you absorb calcium. Excess animal protein promotes calcium loss. Meat-eaters are more likely to get osteoporosis than vegetarians.

Women with osteoporosis are more likely to produce insufficient gastric acid. Calcium absorption needs acid and acid production requires zinc, so eat enough zinc-rich foods. Fats and added sugar reduce acid production.

Calcium may reduce flushes (flashes), and vitamin E may be useful for these and vaginal dryness, especially if your diet also contains plenty of vitamins B and C. Vitamin-A-rich foods help keep mucous membranes healthy. Thiamine and niacin help prevent headaches; riboflavin reduces vaginal itching; B6 helps prevent cramp; and folic acid is necessary for oestrogen formation. Foods rich in calcium and magnesium, and low-protein sources of tryptophan make *depression* less likely. After the menopause the levels of potentially harmful blood fats (LDLs) tend to rise. Keep them low by avoiding saturated fats and eating foods rich in essential fatty acids and vitamin C. Raw fruit and vegetables, nuts, beans and grains have a natural oestrogenic effect. (See **The basic healthy diet** pp. 12-13, **Foods, nutrients, and ailments** pp. 80-2.)

▲ Essential fatty acids; raw fruit and vegetables; nuts, beans, wholegrains; vitamins A, B, C, E, K, and flavonoids; low-protein tryptophan-rich foods; calcium, magnesium, zinc.

▼ Saturated fats; added sugar; meat; coffee, tea, cocoa, and cola.

Mouth ulcers

Thrush and herpes simplex virus ulcers are helped by dietary measures for *infection*. Aphthous ulcers can be associated with *food sensitivity*. Gluten sensitivity is the best known and there may be coincident coeliac disease. Other "culprits" include figs, cheese, tomatoes, walnuts, fruit, azo dyes, and milk. Dietary causes include a deficiency of iron, vitamins B6 or B12, or folic acid.

Diet   Take anti-*Candida* and anti-infection measures (if necessary) and identify "culprit" foods. Eat more garlic and foods rich in iron, vitamins B6 and B12, and folic acid. Cut down on refined carbohydrates. (See **The basic healthy diet** pp. 12-13, **Foods, nutrients, and ailments** pp. 80-2, **The exclusion diet** pp. 91-3.)

▲ Vitamins B6, B12, folic acid; iron; garlic.

▼ "Culprit" foods; refined carbohydrates.

Multiple sclerosis

People with MS tend to have low levels of essential fatty acids and high levels of saturated fats in the lecithin in their myelin sheaths and brain. A high saturated fat diet inhibits the conversion of linoleic acid to prostaglandin E1 in the body, and it is this chemical pathway that may be faulty in MS. One study found that supplements of D-phenylalanine were useful. Phenylalanine is converted into the amino acid tyrosine. Meals high in carbohydrate reduce your blood levels of tyrosine, so try avoiding carbohydrate-rich meals, and having some protein with each meal.

Diet   Eat five or more small meals a day to help combat tiredness. Eat more foods rich in essential fatty acids. These are reported to be 50 times more active in the form of lecithin than in other sources. Some experts recommend a diet in which fruit and vegetables make up 45 per cent of the calories. Make sure you eat enough foods rich in the nutrients needed for myelin production and maintenance, including protein, riboflavin, niacin, vitamins B6, B12, and folic acid; copper, magnesium, manganese, and zinc. Avoid carbohydrate-rich meals. (See **The basic healthy diet** pp. 12-13, **Foods, nutrients, and ailments** pp. 80-2.)

▲ Essential fatty acids and lecithin; oily fish; fresh fruit and vegetables; protein; riboflavin, niacin, vitamins B6, B12, and folic acid; copper, magnesium, manganese, zinc.

▼ Saturated fats.

Nail disorders

Iron-deficiency *anaemia* can cause thin, spoon-shaped nails. A *Candida* nail infection may indicate *Candida* elsewhere (see *Candidiasis*). Alopecia areata can be associated with ridges, pits, and roughness; poor circulation with a loss of nail folds; and zinc deficiency with white spots or brittle nails. Severe iron or protein deficiency make the nail beds white. Split, flaky nails may respond to foods rich in linoleic acid.

Diet   Treat iron deficiency (see *Anaemia*), poor circulation (see *Circulation problems*), or *candidiasis* and identify any "culprit" foods. Eat more protein, zinc, and essential fatty acids if necessary. (See **The basic healthy diet** pp. 12-13, **Foods, nutrients, and ailments** pp. 80-2, **The exclusion diet** pp. 91-3.)

▲ Iron, zinc, essential fatty acids, protein.

▼ "Culprit" foods.

Nausea

There are many causes of nausea and it is sensible to treat the cause rather than merely the sensation.

Diet   Keep your meals small and low in fat. If you are prone to travel sickness, avoid fatty, sugary foods for 24 hours before travelling. Peppermint or chamomile flower tea usually help, and ginger can be excellent. You can sometimes ease pregnancy sickness with raspberry leaf or chamomile tea and foods rich in vitamin B6. (See **The basic healthy diet** pp. 12-13, **Foods, nutrients, and ailments** pp. 80-2.)

▲ Peppermint or chamomile flower tea; fresh or crystallized ginger root. (For pregnancy sickness) vitamin B6; raspberry leaf or chamomile tea.

▼ Large meals; fat; added sugar.

Obesity

If you are 20 per cent above the average weight for your age and height, or 30 per cent above the recommended weight (see p. 89), then you are obese. You are statistically more likely to suffer from a number of diseases or medical complications if you are overweight. These include *arterial disease* (such as heart disease and *high blood pressure*), *arthritis*, *diabetes*, *gallstones*, post-operative complications, hiatus hernia, *cancer* of the breast and uterus, *pregnancy problems*,

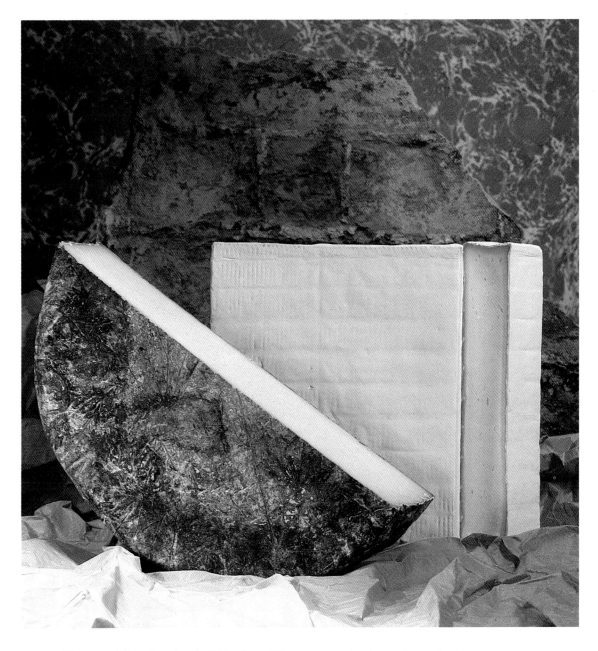

Cheese is rich in vitamins A, B12, D, and E, riboflavin, niacin, calcium, and phosphorus, and contains between 25 and 35 % protein. Making milk into cheese is an excellent way of preserving the goodness of surplus summer supplies. The separation of high- or low-fat milk into curds and whey is hastened by heating and adding animal or vegetable rennet.

varicose veins, menstrual pains, and *constipation*.

Diet Lose excess body fat by eating *the basic healthy diet*, by taking in fewer calories, by exercising more and by dealing with any food sensitivity. One period of exercise raises your metabolic rate for more than a day. If you eat a lot of added sugar, refined cereal, and saturated fat it will be hard for you to lose weight, even if your calorie intake is reasonable. *The basic healthy diet*, high in fibre and low in refined foods, aids weight loss when part of a calorie-controlled diet, as may eating more spices. Eating habits are ingrained from an early age, and food may be associated with feelings of security or insecurity, love, anxiety, and anger. A child from a family with good eating habits that does not use mealtimes as emotional battlegrounds is unlikely to become obese. (See **The basic healthy diet** pp. 12-13, **Foods, nutrients, and ailments** pp. 80-2, **The weight-reducing diet** pp. 87-9.)

Pain

Coffee contains substances that prevent endorphins (your body's natural pain-killers) from working. A diet deficient in copper means that you may not produce enough painkilling enkephalins. Carbohydrates rich in the amino acid tryptophan may raise your pain tolerance because tryptophan enhances the effects of endorphins. Tryptophan-rich foods (see p.56) are only effective if you avoid proteins before and after the meal. Your body's anti-stress hormones depend on adequate amounts of calcium and affect your response to pain.

Diet Avoid coffee and eat enough foods rich in copper and calcium. Tryptophan-rich carbohydrates are helpful, but avoid protein for 90 minutes either side of such a meal. (See **The basic healthy diet** pp. 12-13, **Foods, nutrients and ailments** pp. 80-2.)

▲ Copper, calcium; tryptophan-rich carbohydrates

▼ Coffee; protein (when necessary).

Palpitation

Anxiety is the commonest cause of heart palpitation, but occasionally palpitation indicates heart disease. Caffeine stimulates adrenaline and can cause palpitation. Other causes include *food sensitivity*, deficiencies of thiamine, vitamins B6 and B12, copper, magnesium, and potassium; *anaemia*, and pressure from a hiatus hernia or an overful stomach.

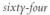

Diet   If you are overanxious (see *Anxiety*), anaemic (see *Anaemia*), or suffer from *low blood sugar* swings, adjust your diet. Reduce your intake of caffeine. If you suspect *food sensitivity*, pinpoint your "culprit" foods. Check you are eating enough thiamine, vitamins B6, and B12, copper, magnesium, and potassium. Deal with a hiatus hernia (see *Acid reflux*) and avoid over-eating and drinking. Fatty foods delay the emptying of the stomach and so may keep it overful for longer. (See **The basic healthy diet** pp. 12-13, **Foods, nutrients, and ailments** pp. 80-2, **The exclusion diet** pp. 91-3.)
▲ Thiamine, vitamins B6, B12; copper, magnesium, potassium, and iron.
▼ "Culprit" foods; refined carbohydrates; large, fatty meals; coffee, tea, cocoa, cola.

Peptic ulcers

Fibre from unrefined carbohydrates and raw fruit and vegetables swells to form a protective gel. Refined carbohydrates make no such gel and so expose the stomach and duodenum linings to stomach acid. Some antacids lead to a deficiency of iron or calcium, while others containing calcium or aluminium can cause excess absorption of these minerals. Do not drink extra milk for ulcers: milk initially lowers acid production, but there is a rapid rebound. Other acid-provoking foods include caffeine-containing drinks. Certain nutrients are protective or healing. A stomach infection with *Helicobacter pylori* may accompany an ulcer and you should eat infection fighting foods.

Diet   Eat more fibre, unrefined carbohydrates, raw fruit and vegetables (especially cabbage) and avoid animal protein, caffeine, alcohol, black pepper, chilli pepper, and refined carbohydrates (especially sugar). Minimize pain with frequent small meals; eat slowly, chew well, and have your meals in a relaxed setting. Take milk or milk products once or twice a day only to avoid repeated acid attack. Eat more foods rich in vitamins A, B6, C, E, and flavonoids, and zinc. If you suspect a *food sensitivity*, identify your "culprit" foods. (See **The basic healthy diet** pp. 12-13, **Foods, nutrients, and ailments** pp. 80-2, **The exclusion diet** pp. 91-3.)
▲ Unrefined carbohydrates; raw fruit and vegetables; vitamins A, B6, C, and E, and flavonoids; zinc; infection-fighting foods.
▼ Refined carbohydrates (especially added sugar); animal protein; coffee, tea, cocoa, cola; alcohol; black pepper; "culprit" foods.

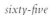

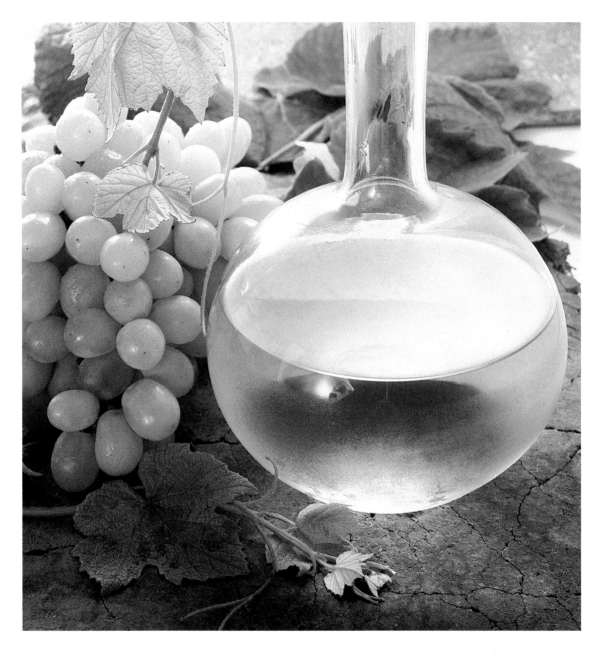

Grapes *contain a form of dietary fibre called pectin, which helps lower low-density lipoprotein (LDL) cholesterol in the blood. Grapes are a good source of biotin and contain vitamin C and small amounts of many minerals that are also present in wine. The sweetness of grapes is due to fruit sugar, which is twice as sweet, weight for weight, as most other sugars.*

Period (menstrual) problems

Eating a lot of meat and being deficient in vitamins A, B6, and C, flavonoids, iron, and zinc can lead to heavy periods. Flavonoids and vitamin C help prevent heavy bleeding. A deficiency of calcium, magnesium, zinc, or essential fatty acids, a *food sensitivity* or a *Candida* infection can cause period pain. Vitamins B6, and E, and niacin are vital for a healthy uterus and ovaries.

Diet For heavy periods, eat more raw fruit and vegetables, especially citrus fruit with the pith on, and foods rich in vitamins A and B6, iron, and zinc. For period pains eat foods rich in calcium, magnesium, zinc, vitamins B, C and E and flavonoids, and essential fatty acids; eat less saturated fat, and take raspberry leaf tea for three days before your period is due and ginger, cramp bark and caraway seed teas during your period. If you suspect a *food sensitivity* identify your "culprit" foods. Use the anti-*Candida* diet (see *Candidiasis*) for a *Candida* infection. For all period problems eat enough foods rich in niacin, vitamin B6, and E. (See **The basic healthy diet** pp. 12-13, **Foods, nutrients and ailments** pp. 80-2, **The exclusion diet** pp. 91-3.)

▲ (For heavy periods) raw fruit (especially citrus) and vegetables; vitamins A and B6; iron, zinc. (For period pains) essential fatty acids; vitamins B, C and E and flavonoids; calcium, magnesium, zinc; raspberry leaf, ginger root, cramp bark, and caraway seed teas. (For all period problems) niacin, vitamin B6, E.

▼ (For period pains) saturated fat; "culprit" foods.

Physical performance problems

Diet Avoid *low blood sugar* swings. A high-carbohydrate diet increases glycogen stores. A high-fat diet does the opposite, while high-protein diets can lead to potassium deficiency with cramps or even an irregular heartbeat. Alcohol can reduce performance. Take fruit and vegetable juices to replace lost minerals, and eat foods rich in potassium (for glycogen formation, and for lessening the risk of cramp and muscle injury); magnesium (for co-ordination and speed of reaction); the B vitamins (for replacing loss in sweat and urine); calcium and iron (for optimum performance). (See **The basic healthy diet** pp. 12-13, **Foods, nutrients, and ailments** pp. 80-2.)

▲ Unrefined carbohydrates; fruit and vegetable juices; vitamin B; calcium, iron, potassium, magnesium.

▼ Refined carbohydrates; protein; excess alcohol and fat.

Pregnancy problems

Low birth weight, pre-eclampsia, *anaemia*, miscarriage, malformations, and premature labour can all be influenced by what you eat.

Diet Too much or too little food can lead to problems, as can deficiencies of individual nutrients. Eat nutritious foods and avoid wasting your intake on "empty" calories. Being overweight before pregnancy leads to a high risk of pre-eclampsia. But do not start a weight-reducing diet while pregnant, just avoid "empty" calories.

Eat plenty of foods rich in vitamins A, B6, folic acid, pantothenic acid, C, E, and flavonoids, iron, manganese, zinc, and essential fatty acids. Zinc deficiency is frequently found in mothers of stillborn babies, and low zinc levels have been associated with premature births and certain malformations. Women with pre-eclampsia may have low levels of vitamin B6 or may be getting insufficient calcium. Foods rich in magnesium may help prevent pre-eclampsia as well. Low vitamin E levels may lead to threatened or recurrent miscarriage. Foods rich in calcium, magnesium, and essential fatty acids may help prevent premature labour. A folic-acid deficiency can cause low birth weight and possibly certain malformations. Flavonoids may help prevent miscarriage and pre-term labour. Avoid alcohol because there is no known safe amount to drink – excessive alcohol makes low birth weight more likely and it may also hinder conception. Never eat undercooked meat because of the risk of toxoplasmosis, an infection that could harm your baby. Avoid soft cheese and poorly stored or re-heated cook-chilled food.

Before labour begins, and in early labour, eat high-fibre foods, low in added sugar, to maintain your blood sugar levels and reduce weakness and fatigue. Raspberry leaf tea may help make your labour easier. Chamomile and raspberry leaf tea, and foods rich in vitamin B6 help alleviate morning sickness, and lime blossom tea is useful for raised blood pressure. (See **The basic healthy diet** pp. 12-13, **Foods, nutrients, and ailments** pp. 80-2.)

▲ (For pre-eclampsia) vitamin B6; calcium, magnesium; lime blossom tea. (For miscarriage) vitamin E, and flavonoids; zinc; raspberry leaf tea. (For malformations) folic acid; zinc. (For pre-term birth) flavonoids; calcium, magnesium, zinc; essential fatty acids. (For low birth weight) folic acid.

▼ (For malformations and low birth weight) alcohol.

Pre-menstrual syndrome

Diet If you suffer from *anxiety*, mood swings, irritability, insomnia, and tension (PMS "A"), eat more foods rich in vitamins B (especially B6) and E, and magnesium. If you have *constipation*, increase your fibre intake. It may help to reduce dairy foods and added sugar. If you have weight gain, breast tenderness and swelling, and swelling of your ankles, fingers, and abdomen (PMS "H"), cut down on salt for three days before your symptoms usually begin. Eat more foods rich in vitamins B6, E, and magnesium, and cut added sugar and caffeine down. Breast tenderness may reflect a need for more essential fatty acids. Vitamin B6, magnesium and zinc enhance the use of linoleic acid, but alcohol and saturated fats may hinder its metabolism. If you crave sweet things and have tiredness, an increased appetite, dizziness, palpitations, faintness, and *headaches* (PMS "C"), eat more foods rich in vitamins A, B6, and E, chromium, and magnesium. Reduce your intake of refined carbohydrates and saturated fats. If you suffer from *depression*, tearfulness, *confusion*, forgetfulness, and *insomnia* (PMS "D") eat more foods rich in thiamine, vitamins B6, C, and E, iron, magnesium, and zinc. If you get *acne* before a period, foods rich in zinc may help. Alcohol tends to aggravate PMS. Some women have a *food sensitivity* that increases their symptoms – so try to identify any "culprit" foods. *Candida* infection (see *Candidiasis*) makes PMS worse. Tryptophan–rich, low-protein foods (see p.56) may help if you suffer from *depression* and crave carbohydrates. (See **The basic healthy diet** pp. 12-13, **Foods, nutrients, and ailments** pp. 80-2, **The exclusion diet** pp. 91-3.)

▲ (For PMS "A") vitamins B and E; magnesium; fibre. (For PMS "H") essential fatty acids; vitamins B6 and E; magnesium, zinc. (For PMS "C") vitamins A, B6, and E; chromium, magnesium. (For PMS "D") thiamine, vitamins B6, C, and E; iron, magnesium, zinc. (For all PMS) vitamins B6 and E; magnesium.

▼ (For PMS "A") dairy food; added sugar. (For PMS "H") salt; added sugar; alcohol; saturated fats; coffee, tea, cocoa, cola. (For PMS "C") saturated fat; refined carbohydrates (especially added sugar). (For all PMS) alcohol; "culprit" foods.

Prostate problems

Diet Eat less meat, dairy food, caffeine, and refined carbohydrates. Lose weight, if necessary. Eat more foods rich in zinc,

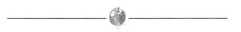

magnesium, selenium, vitamins C and E, fibre, and essential fatty acids (especially from vegetable lecithin). Eat a variety of vegetable proteins to give you enough of the amino acids glycine, alanine, and glutamic acid, thought to be helpful for prostate enlargement. Brewer's yeast, lentils, nuts, and corn are good sources. Zinc-rich pumpkin seeds may help, too. (See **The basic healthy diet** pp. 12-13, **Foods, nutrients, and ailments** pp. 80-2, **The weight-reducing diet** pp. 87-9.)

▲ Essential fatty acids; fibre; vitamins C and E; magnesium, selenium, zinc; vegetable proteins.

▼ Meat; dairy food; coffee, tea, cocoa, and cola; refined carbohydrates (especially added sugar).

Psoriasis

The excessive turnover of skin leads to a need for more folic acid and magnesium. Many sufferers produce little stomach acid.

Diet It may help to cut animal protein down, or out. Eat more foods rich in folic acid, vitamins A and E, zinc, and the essential fatty acids. Reduce animal fat, which interferes with the utilization of essential fatty acids. Eat raw fruit and vegetables. (See **The basic healthy diet** pp. 12-13, **Foods, nutrients, and ailments** pp. 80-2.)

▲ Essential fatty acids; raw fruit and vegetables; vitamins A, E, and folic acid; zinc.

▼ Animal protein and fat.

Rheumatism

Diet Zinc may help stiff or aching joints, and foods rich in vitamin B6 may ease tenosynovitis. Eat more vitamins B6, B12, C, D, flavonoids, calcium, and magnesium. Garlic, feverfew (do not eat for more than 14 consecutive days), celery and celery seed, asparagus, nettle and marjoram teas are soothing. Consume more raw fruit and vegetables and less alcohol, caffeine-containing drinks, added sugar, and animal protein. A *food sensitivity* might cause joint pains. (See **The basic healthy diet** pp. 12-13, **Foods, nutrients, and ailments** pp. 80-2, **The exclusion diet** pp. 91-3.)

▲ Vitamins B6, B12, C, D, and the flavonoids; calcium, magnesium, zinc; garlic, feverfew, celery; celery seed, asparagus; nettle and marjoram teas; raw fruit and vegetables.

▼ Alcohol; coffee, tea, cocoa, cola; added sugar; animal protein.

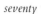

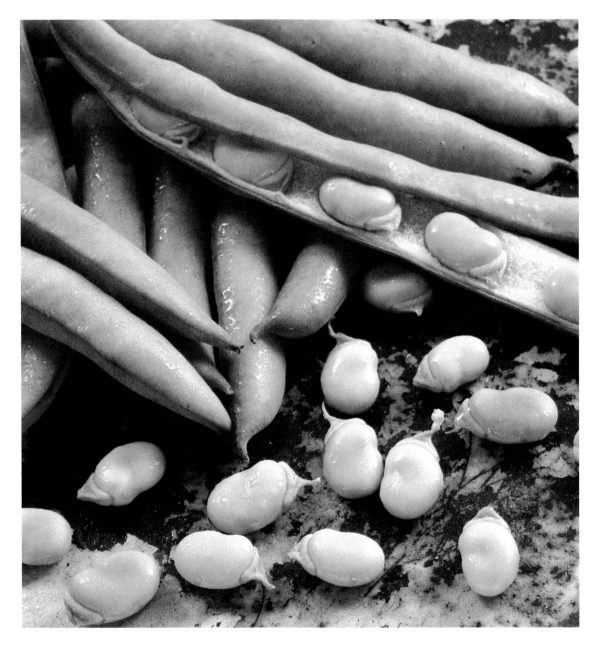

Broad beans are surprisingly richer in protein than meat, fish, and eggs. Their "lente" carbohydrates are absorbed especially slowly, which helps steady the blood sugar level. This makes beans a very useful food for diabetics. Their water-soluble fibre can help lower dangerously high levels of low-density lipoprotein (LDL) cholesterol in the blood.

Rickets

Rickets is caused by a lack of vitamin D, obtained from the diet, and from the action of ultra-violet light from sunshine on the skin.

Diet Eat more foods rich in calcium and vitamin D. If you are breast-feeding, help protect your baby by eating plenty of calcium- and vitamin-D-rich foods. Rickets is more common among inner-city children, vegan children, and in Asians living in cold, cloudy climates. In the last example this occurs partly because the dough used to make chappatis is unleavened. Thus phytates in the wheat fibre are present in higher amounts than in leavened bread and these reduce the absorption of calcium from the gut. Daylight in colder, more northerly climates is relatively ineffective in producing vitamin D, so dietary supplies of vitamin D are particularly important. (See **The basic healthy diet** pp. 12-13, **Foods, nutrients, and ailments** pp. 80-2.)

▲ Vitamin D; calcium.

▼ Unleavened bread.

Schizophrenia

There is an increasing amount of research into the diet as part of the treatment of schizophrenia, but there is no evidence that the diet plays an important causative role. Some sufferers have a *food sensitivity*. One in two sufferers has defective eyesight. Deficiencies of vitamin C, folic acid, manganese, and zinc can cause a schizophrenic-type episode or an exacerbation of chronic schizophrenia, as can folic acid or copper poisoning. Nutritional deficiencies of vitamins B and C, chromium, magnesium, manganese, and zinc are widespread. Some sufferers lose large amounts of zinc in urine. Certain brain neurotransmitters are altered in schizophrenia, and the diet is known to affect these. One in two sufferers lacks histamine and some have an excess of dopamine.

Diet Eat *the basic healthy diet*, rich in niacin, vitamins B1, B6, B12, folic acid, and C, as well as essential fatty acids, chromium, magnesium, manganese, and zinc. Cut down on your caffeine and meat intake. If you suspect a *food sensitivity*, pinpoint your "culprit" foods. (See **The basic healthy diet** pp. 12-13, **Foods, nutrients, and ailments** pp. 80-2, **The exclusion diet** pp. 91-3.)

▲ Essential fatty acids; niacin, vitamins B1, B6, B12, folic acid, and C; chromium, magnesium, manganese, zinc.

▼ Coffee, tea, cocoa, cola; "culprit" foods; meat.

Sex drive problems

The typical westernized refined diet probably accounts for many people having a low sex drive.

Diet   Eat plenty of foods rich in vitamins A and E, magnesium, manganese, zinc, and vegetable protein. These nutrients are important for sex hormone production and healthy reproductive organs. Eat plenty of raw fruit and vegetables. Alcohol may make you feel sexy temporarily, but does nothing for performance. (See **The basic healthy diet** pp. 12-13, **Foods, nutrients, and ailments** pp. 80-2.)

▲ Vegetable protein; raw fruit and vegetables; vitamins A and E; magnesium, manganese, zinc.

Short-sightedness

A short-sighted (myopic) person cannot focus an image on the retina. Short sight is more likely if you eat poorly. Some people manage to alleviate or control short sight by adjusting their diet.

Diet Eat more foods rich in vitamins B6, C, E, and folic acid, calcium, and chromium. Folic acid is probably the most important nutrient for the prevention and reversal of short sight. Fresh, raw, green leafy vegetables are the best source (folic acid is easily destroyed by heat) and also contain vitamin C and calcium. Chromium is generally found in high levels in naturally sweet foods. A highly refined diet, containing added sugar and meat, may be deficient in chromium and have an excess of vanadium. Alcohol may make your eyesight temporarily worse and *lead poisoning* makes short sight more likely. (See **The basic healthy diet** pp. 12-13, **Foods, nutrients, and ailments** pp. 80-2.)

▲ Vitamins B6, C, E, and folic acid; calcium, chromium.
▼ Added sugar; meat; alcohol.

Smoking

Smokers have a small appetite, and a low "junk food margin". You need one and a half times the vitamin C of a non-smoker because each cigarette destroys 25mg of the vitamin. Vitamin C and selenium help neutralize toxins such as cadmium that are absorbed from the smoke. Cadmium is a zinc antagonist, so you need more zinc. Smoking makes you more prone to illness and decreases magnesium levels. You may be at risk of a vitamin B6 deficiency

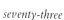

and you are well advised to increase the amount of calcium and vitamin B12 in your diet. Smoking speeds up caffeine metabolism, so you may need more and more coffee. If you are breast-feeding, the nicotine may decrease the amount of milk you make. Smoking can inhibit pancreatic enzymes, which can lead to poor digestion.

Diet Eat more foods rich in vitamins B (especially B6 and B12) and C; calcium, magnesium, selenium, and zinc. Watch for an increasing need for caffeine. If you are trying to cut down on smoking, you may find sunflower seeds (containing oils and B vitamins) have a soothing effect. (See **The basic healthy diet** pp. 12-13, **Foods, nutrients, and ailments** pp. 80-2.)

▲ Vitamins B6, B12, and C; calcium, magnesium, selenium, zinc; sunflower seeds.

Stress

Stress increases the requirements for certain nutrients because the body uses or loses more when it is under pressure. It also makes *food sensitivity* more likely.

Diet Avoid refined carbohydrates, and eat more fibre-rich foods. The flavonoids in citrus fruit pith are helpful. You need more foods rich in vitamin B (especially riboflavin), C and E, calcium, magnesium, phosphorus, potassium, zinc, and essential fatty acids. Make meals relaxed occasions to help digestion. Eating little and often helps your body absorb more nutrients. If you suspect a *food sensitivity*, identify your "culprit" foods. Avoid caffeine-containing drinks. (See **The basic healthy diet** pp. 12-13, **Foods, nutrients, and ailments** pp. 80-2, **The exclusion diet** pp. 91-3.)

▲ Essential fatty acids; fibre; vitamins B, C, E, and the flavonoids; calcium, magnesium, phosphorus, potassium, zinc.

▼ Refined carbohydrates (especially added sugar); "culprit" foods; coffee, tea, cocoa, cola.

Taste loss

Many people are unable to taste their food as well as they should and this often accompanies a reduction in their ability to smell. The loss of the senses of taste and smell is one of the first signs of zinc deficiency.

Diet Eat more foods rich in zinc. (See **The basic healthy diet** pp. 12-13, **Foods, nutrients, and ailments** pp. 80-2.)

▲ Zinc.

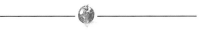

Thinness

Worldwide, the most common cause for being underweight is malnutrition. This is primarily a problem of developing countries, but it exists in westernized countries, too. The medically accepted range of normal weight for a person of given height, age, and build is very wide (see p.89). Most experts consider it healthier to be of average, or below average, weight. If you feel you are too thin you need to find ways of increasing your appetite (see *Appetite loss*), and digest and use your food as well as you can.

Diet You will digest and absorb nutrients better if you eat several small meals a day, rather than a few large ones. Avoid a long gap over night by having a snack before bed. It is particularly important to spread your protein intake throughout the day, since your body will make better use of it. Try to make your meals relaxed to aid digestion. Choose nutrient-packed foods and avoid "empty" calories, and caffeine-containing drinks. (See **The basic healthy diet** pp. 12-13, **Foods, nutrients, and ailments** pp. 80-2.)

▲ Nutrient-rich foods.

▼ Refined carbohydrates; animal fat; coffee, tea, cocoa, cola.

Tiredness

Tiredness may be a warning that you are unwell or overdoing things. A refined diet may lack necessary nutrients and encourage *low blood sugar* swings. Undue tiredness can be caused by a *food sensitivity*, the *pre-menstrual syndrome* and *anaemia*.

Diet Eat more foods rich in vitamins B (especially pantothenic acid, B12, and folic acid), C and E, iron, magnesium, and potassium. Choose more protein-containing foods from vegetable sources and cut down refined carbohydrates. Fibre-rich foods help avoid *low blood sugar* swings. Take lime flower, elderflower, and chamomile teas instead of caffeine-containing drinks. Eat plenty of foods rich in essential fatty acids, but less total fat. A day on a fruit and vegetable juice *semi-fast* may help. (See **The basic healthy diet** pp. 12-13, **Foods, nutrients, and ailments** pp. 80-2, **The semi-fast diet** p. 90.)

▲ Fibre; essential fatty acids; raw fruit and vegetables; vitamins B, C, and E; iron, magnesium, potassium, vegetable protein; lime flower, elderflower, and chamomile teas.

▼ "Empty" calories; refined carbohydrates; coffee, tea, cocoa, cola; total fat.

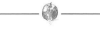

Tooth decay

Teeth gradually become coated with plaque, which is formed from food residue and bacteria. Sugars are present in the mouth from carbohydrates. The bacteria in the sticky layer of plaque feed on these sugars and release acid, which eats into dental enamel. If the acid attack is frequent enough, or the sugars are in the mouth for long enough, and if the acid level rises too high, cavities form and tooth decay results. Children are more prone to decay than adults and some children have more dental decay (caries) than others. A diet high in refined carbohydrates increases the thickness of the plaque. Foods and drinks containing added sugar are the most cariogenic. An optimum intake of fluoride from food and drinking water may minimize the risk of decay.

Diet   Follow meals containing added sugar with nuts or cheese to counteract acidity. If you eat sugary food or drinks, or sticky foods such as dried fruits, clean your teeth afterwards. (See **The basic healthy diet** pp. 12-13, **Foods, nutrients, and ailments** pp. 80-2.)

▲ Fluoride (if necessary).

▼ Sugary and sticky foods and drinks between meals.

Urinary tract infection

Infection in the kidneys (pyelonephritis) or bladder (cystitis) is more common in people eating a poor diet. Certain foods encourage infection by altering the acidity of the urine.

Diet   Choose an anti-*infection* diet. Drink plenty of water (or home-made lemon barley water) to flush your urinary tract through and reduce the burning. Start with 550ml (1pt/2 large cupfuls) of water and follow with 275ml (tpt/1 large cupful) every 20 minutes for three hours. Add one teaspoonful of sodium bicarbonate every hour to make your urine more alkaline. Eat fewer "acid-producing" foods (see pp.80-2), and more fruit and vegetables to alkalinize your urine. Eat more vitamin-E-rich foods to protect your urinary tract and decrease the amount of animal fat. Treat any *Candida* infection (see *Candidiasis*) and if you suspect a *food sensitivity*, identify your "culprit" foods. Avoid caffeine-containing drinks and alcohol. Raw garlic several times a day and asparagus are helpful, as are cranberry juice and teas made with parsley, feverfew, meadowsweet, and borage. Two days on a *semi-fast*, followed by a day on raw fruit and vegetables helps most people. (See **The basic healthy diet** pp. 12-13, **Foods, nutrients, and ailments** pp. 80-2,

The semi-fast diet p. 90, **The exclusion diet** pp. 91-3.)

▲ Water; bicarbonate of soda; fruit and vegetables; lemon barley water; vitamin E; garlic; asparagus; cranberry juice; parsley, feverfew, meadowsweet, and borage teas.

▼ Animal protein; cereals; animal fat; "culprit" foods; coffee, tea, cocoa, and cola.

Varicose veins

You can help prevent varicose veins by eating a healthy diet. If you are overweight you are more likely to suffer. Constipation can cause back pressure in the leg veins from the loaded bowel pressing on the pelvic veins and from straining to pass bowel motions.

Diet Lose weight, if necessary, and avoid *constipation*. Eat more foods rich in vitamin C and flavonoids to strengthen your veins. Vitamin B6-rich foods may help if you are pregnant. (See **The basic healthy diet** pp. 12-13, **Foods, nutrients, and ailments** pp. 80-2, **The weight-reducing diet** pp. 87-9.)

▲ Fibre; vitamins B6, C, and flavonoids; water.

▼ Refined carbohydrates.

Wind (gas)

Wind (gas) results from swallowing air; from poor digestion; from fermentation caused by bacteria or *Candida* (see *Candidiasis*) in the stomach or gut; from certain foods or carbonated drinks; or from the *irritable bowel syndrome*.

Diet Chew well and try not to talk while eating. Bacterial or *Candida* overgrowth can be caused by a poor diet, antibiotics, or too little gastric acid. Treat *constipation*, and if you suspect a *food sensitivity* identify your "culprit" foods. Fatty foods, raw vegetables and fruit, added sugar, an excess of high-fibre foods, caffeine-containing drinks, and pulses (beans and peas) make some people windy (gassy). Others suffer if they eat starchy food with protein. Soak pulses (beans and peas) before boiling. Pawpaw, pineapple, angelica root tea, and mustard or dill seeds can help. Both breast- and bottle-fed babies may suffer; seek professional advice. (See **The basic healthy diet** pp. 12-13, **Foods, nutrients, and ailments** pp. 80-2, **The exclusion diet** pp. 91-3.)

▲ Pawpaw; pineapple; mustard and dill seeds; angelica root tea.

▼ Meat; refined carbohydrates (especially added sugar); pulses (beans and peas); "culprit" foods; fats; coffee, tea, cocoa, cola.

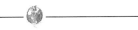

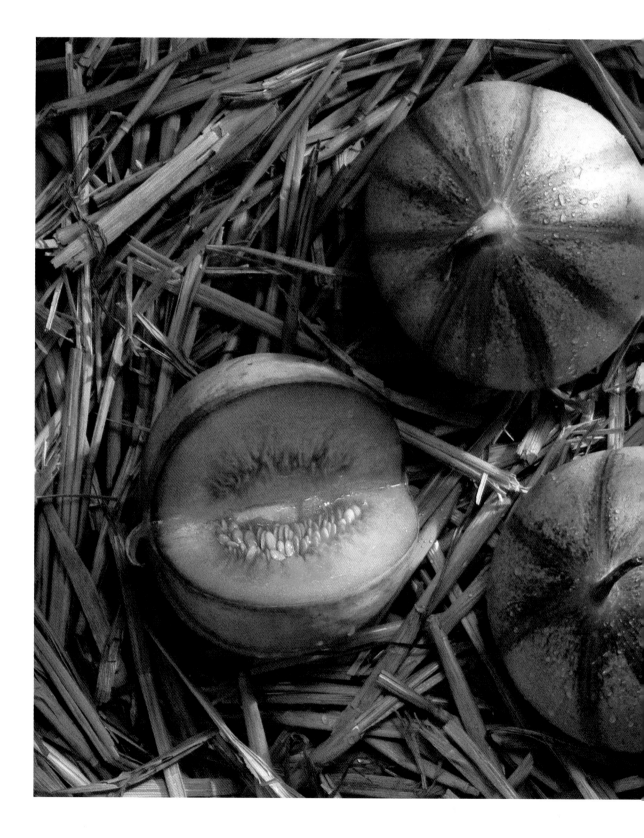

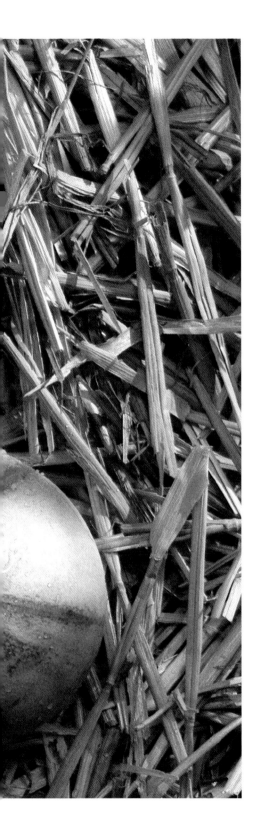

THE SPECIAL DIETS

No one but you can choose whether or not to opt for the way of health. A lifetime of treating yourself well by eating nutritious and lovingly chosen food lowers your risk of many common ailments, including some chronic degenerative conditions such as arterial disease.

Our term "diet" means "a way of eating". The word stems from the Greek word *diaita*, meaning a way of life. The way of life you choose, along with the food you eat, determine how well you are. However, it may be that you have only recently learnt how to care for yourself through what you eat. This chapter shows you how to embark on eating plans to help lower your fat intake (especially saturated fat), reduce salt levels in your diet, reduce your weight, rest your bowel by eating lightly for a short time, and pinpoint individual foods that may be giving you problems caused by food sensitivity. Once you begin to feel better, you can nearly always slowly adapt to *the basic healthy diet* as a permanent way of eating. A return to your old ways would simply mean a recurrence of your problems at a later period in your life. (The diets are preceded by a self-help chart **Foods, nutrients, and ailments**.)

Foods, nutrients, and ailments

Foods (columns): Milk, Cheeses, Eggs, Egg yolk, Fish, Tinned fish, Fatty fish, Shellfish, Meat, Offal (organ meat), Chicken, Black pudding, Haggis, Wholegrain rice, Wholegrain cereals, Beans/peas, Soya beans, Lentils, Peanuts, Broccoli, Lettuce, Spinach, Parsley

Nutrients (rows): Calcium, Chromium, Copper, Iodine, Iron, Magnesium, Manganese, Phosphorus, Potassium, Selenium, Sulphur, Vanadium, Zinc, Vitamin A, Thiamine, Riboflavin, Niacin, Pantothenic acid, Vitamin B6, Vitamin B12, Folic acid, Vitamin C, Vitamin D, Vitamin E, Vitamin K, Flavonoids, Fibre, Essential fatty acids, Acid-producing foods, Alkali-producing foods

Ailments (lower columns): Poor concentration, Depression, Insomnia, Tiredness, Numbness/tingling, Clumsiness, Dizziness, Headaches, Dislike of noise, Deafness, Ringing in ears, Taste loss, Poor sense of smell, Poor night vision, Dislike of light, Irritability, Anxiety, Restlessness, Heart racing, Irregular heartbeat, Shortness of breath, Angina, Diarrhoea

This chart (pp. 80-3) gives a selection of foods, nutrients, and ailments. To find out what nutrients a food contains, read down until you see a green triangle, then left. To find out what foods *(continued)*

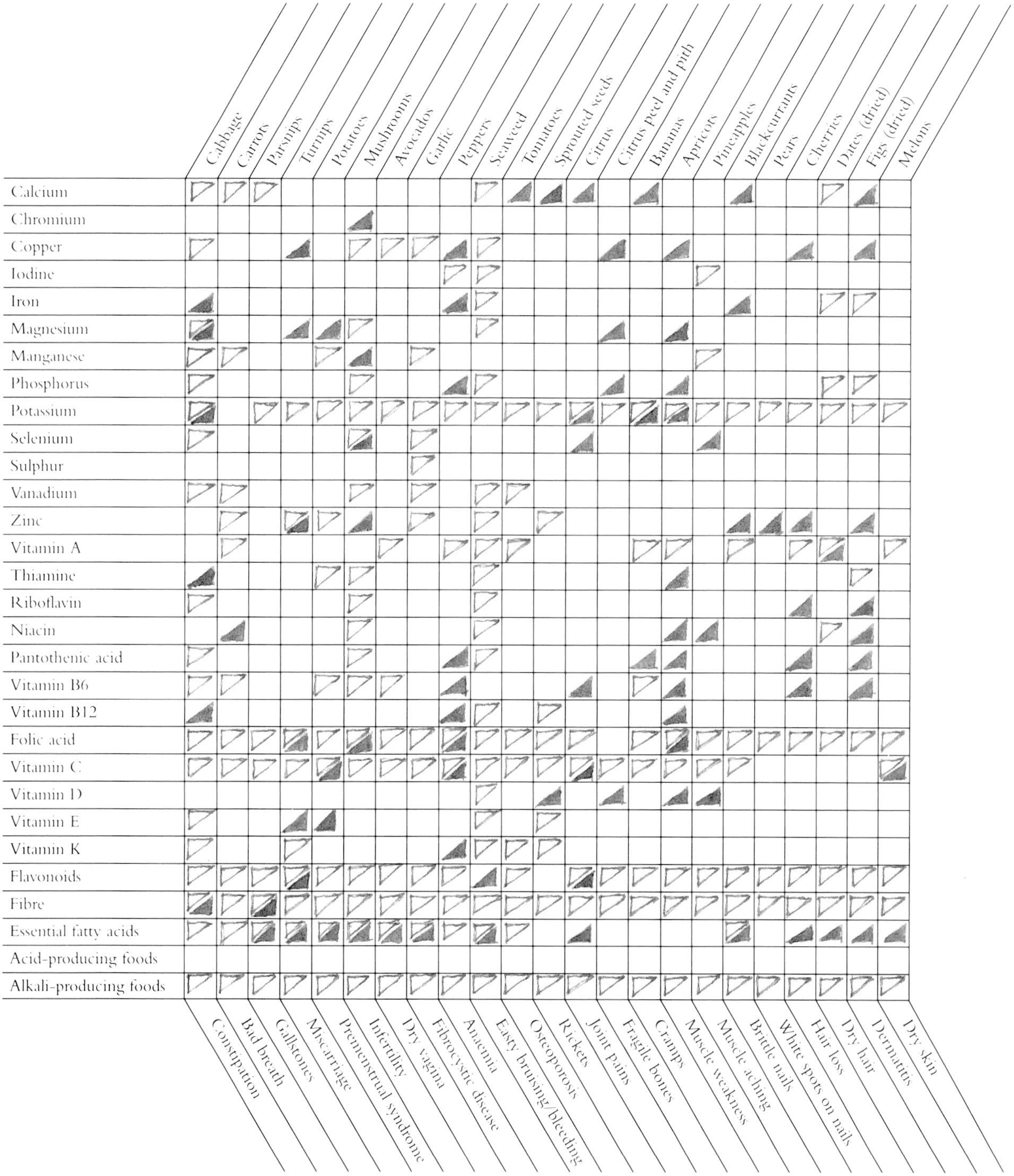
Cabbage
Carrots
Parsnips
Turnips
Potatoes
Mushrooms
Avocados
Garlic
Peppers
Seaweed
Tomatoes
Sprouted seeds
Citrus
Citrus peel and pith
Bananas
Apricots
Pineapples
Blackcurrants
Pears
Cherries
Dates (dried)
Figs (dried)
Melons
Calcium
Chromium
Copper
Iodine
Iron
Magnesium
Manganese
Phosphorus
Potassium
Selenium
Sulphur
Vanadium
Zinc
Vitamin A
Thiamine
Riboflavin
Niacin
Pantothenic acid
Vitamin B6
Vitamin B12
Folic acid
Vitamin C
Vitamin D
Vitamin E
Vitamin K
Flavonoids
Fibre
Essential fatty acids
Acid-producing foods
Alkali-producing foods
Constipation
Bad breath
Gallstones
Miscarriage
Premenstrual syndrome
Infertility
Dry vagina
Fibrocystic disease
Anaemia
Easty bruising/bleeding
Osteoporosis
Rickets
Joint pains
Fragile bones
Cramps
Muscle weakness
Muscle aching
Brittle nails
White spots on nails
Hair loss
Dry hair
Dermatitis
Dry skin

contain a certain nutrient, read across from the nutrients first, then up. To find out what nutrient deficiencies cause certain ailments, read up first, until you see an orange triangle, then left.

Food columns (left to right): Strawberries, Grapes, Plums, Seeds, Sunflower seeds, Nuts, Hard water, Black pepper, Wheatgerm, Yeast, Yeast extract, Molasses, Chocolate, Cocoa, Iodized salt, Tea, Root ginger, Paprika pepper, Fermented soya, Fermented foods, Butter, Polyunsat. margarines, Cold-pressed veg. oils

Nutrient rows (top to bottom): Calcium, Chromium, Copper, Iodine, Iron, Magnesium, Manganese, Phosphorus, Potassium, Selenium, Sulphur, Vanadium, Zinc, Vitamin A, Thiamine, Riboflavin, Niacin, Pantothenic acid, Vitamin B6, Vitamin B12, Folic acid, Vitamin C, Vitamin D, Vitamin E, Vitamin K, Bioflavonoids, Fibre, Essential fatty acids, Acid-producing foods, Alkali-producing foods

Ailment columns (bottom, left to right): Lip cracking, Lip dryness/burning, Acne, Dandruff, Gooseflesh, Gum disease, Tooth decay, Night sweats, Diabetes, Blood sugar swings, Poor immunity, Weight loss, Difficulty swallowing, Sore tongue, Feeling cold, Abnormal thirst, Poor wound healing, Burning feet, Dry eyes, Conjunctivitis, Poor growth, Appetite loss, Nausea

The low-fat diet

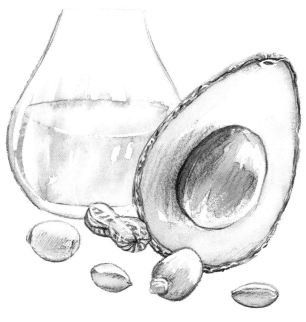

About 30 per cent of the calories in *the basic healthy diet* are fat, and only 10 per cent of this is saturated fat. Many people eating a westernized diet eat too much fat – especially the saturated kind, and these high levels have been linked to several common health problems.

It is sensible to cut down your saturated fat intake if you are suffering from *arterial disease* (including *high blood pressure* or angina), and if you have had a stroke or a heart attack. It may also help if you have *circulation problems*; if you have *gallstones* and are intolerant of fatty foods; if you have continuing diarrhoea after an attack of *gastroenteritis*; or if you have hepatitis. Cutting down your total fat intake reduces the risk of *cancer* of the breast, uterus, gallbladder, and colon.

Reducing fat intake is often hard. Concentrate on cutting down the amount of saturated fat you eat to about 10 per cent of your total calories. Saturated fat predominates in animal fat (fat on and in meat, poultry, eggs, milk, cheese, yoghurt, butter, suet, lard, and dripping) and hard margarines and cooking fats. It is unusual for anyone to eat too much unsaturated fat. This is found in many vegetable oils and soft margarines, fatty fish, nuts, and seeds, as well as in smaller amounts in wholegrain cereals and some vegetables and legumes.

As you eat less saturated fat, the proportion of unsaturated fats in your diet automatically increases. This is good and may be medically helpful, for instance, in preventing or treating *high blood pressure* and *arterial disease*, *arthritis*, and *gallstones*. If you have high blood levels of cholesterol, reduce your intake of saturated fats. This is usually much more helpful in lowering blood cholesterol levels than eating less cholesterol. However, a minority of people need to lower their cholesterol intake. The main sources are eggs and meat.

Avoid buying high-fat foods

- *Buy white meat (poultry or fish) instead of red meat.*
- *Choose lean meat and mince.*
- *Do not buy sausages, sausage meat, luncheon meat, or liver sausage.*
- *Avoid cream, full-fat yoghurt, and cheese (except 1% or less low-fat cottage). Curd cheese, quark, or proprietary lower-fat cheeses are acceptable.*
- *Buy semi-skimmed or skimmed milk instead of whole milk.*
- *Avoid cakes, biscuits, pastry, confectionery, and desserts made with fat or shortening.*
- *Choose vinegar, low- or non-fat yoghurt, or lemon juice for salad dressing, not high-fat dressings.*
- *Buy a cis-linoleic-acid-based margarine and cut down the amount you use.*
- *"Low-fat" margarine is a mixture of fat and water. It contains less fat than other margarines, but it still contains a lot of fat and this may be saturated.*

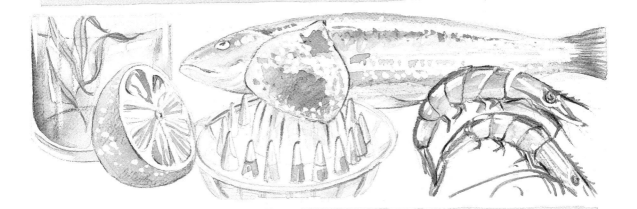

Prepare food wisely

- *Brush the frying pan with a very little oil or use a non-stick pan.*
- *Avoid deep-fat frying.*
- *Remove fat from meat or poultry before cooking.*
- *Stand meat on a rack for grilling, baking, or roasting.*
- *Bake meat, poultry, or fish in a terracotta pot to avoid adding fat.*
- *Skim fat from casseroles or soups while cooking. Use kitchen paper to blot up small amounts from the surface.*
- *Let a casserole cool, then remove solidified fat from top.*
- *Thicken gravies, and sauces with cornflour or arrowroot, instead of a roux.*
- *Reduce your spreading fat and cooking fat or oil. Keep to 3 teaspoonsful a day if you need to be strict.*

Minimize your fat intake as you eat

● Spread butter or margarine very thinly. It spreads more easily when not used straight from the refrigerator.
● Remove skin from poultry.
● Cut the visible fat from meat.
● If you do eat anything fried, drain it on absorbent kitchen paper first.

Be a more creative cook

Most people on a high-fat, westernized diet do not find it hard to cut down their fat intake a little. However, once you start cutting the fat content of your diet down to 30 per cent of your total calorie intake, you may find that your food tastes different. Be creative with flavourings and experiment with herbs and spices. These are widely used by populations eating a healthy "low-fat" diet.

Check your vitamins

When you cut down your total and saturated fat, eat a healthy diet to provide all the fat-soluble vitamins A, D, E, and K you need. A variety of whole grains, yellow, green, and orange fruits and vegetables, green leafy vegetables, peas and beans, nuts, and seeds, with some cold water, fatty fish, and limited amounts of dairy produce and eggs, gives you a vitamin-rich diet.

Make up for the lost fat

Unless you also want to lose weight, make up for the loss of calories resulting from the reduction of fat in your diet by eating more fruit, vegetables, and wholegrain cereals.

REMEMBER

Certain fats are a vital component of the diet. These are the essential fatty acids.

The low-salt diet

This diet helps *high blood pressure, kidney stones*, and water retention. "Salt" implies "sodium", present in: brine (sodium chloride); sodium bicarbonate; baking powder; monosodium glutamate; sodium alginate (in cake mixes and milk shakes); preservatives (such as sodium benzoate and sodium nitrate or nitrite); the anti-oxidant sodium ascorbate; acidity regulators (in pickles and bread); sodium saccharine, and "sodium" additives in sweets, biscuits, cakes, dessert mixes, jellies, pie fillings, jams, mock and whipping cream, cream substitute, cheese, canned fruit and vegetables, self-raising flour, soft drinks and wine.

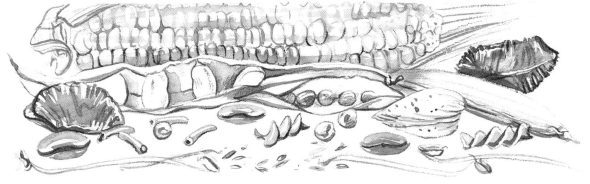

To reduce the amount of sodium or "salt" you eat:

● *Avoid: bacon, ham, sausages, beefburgers, corned beef; salted fish; bread, cereals and cereal flour products (unless without salt, baking powder, or sodium additives); canned and frozen vegetables; butter and margarine with added salt; milk; cheese; ice-cream and milk shakes; stock cubes; yeast extract; salted snacks; popcorn; peanut butter; sauces; mustard; pickles; canned or packet soups; carbonated drinks; and cocoa.*

● *Read the labels of processed foods and avoid any with added salt.*
● *Do not wash or cook vegetables in salted water.*
● *Do not be tempted to add salt, baking powder, monosodium glutamate, or bicarbonate of soda to any recipes.*
● *Do not add salt to the food on your plate.*
● *Do not eat beetroot, carrots, celery, spinach, or sauerkraut.*
● *Eat more vegetable protein and less animal protein.*

The weight-reducing diet

Losing weight is the first line of treatment for many conditions, and many people say that being lighter makes them feel fitter. Perhaps the greatest problem with weight loss is that it is usually difficult to keep the weight off once you have lost it. Over the years there have been many "miracle" diets, all claiming to have found the answer to weight loss. But experience has proved that the only sure way of arriving at and maintaining your target ideal weight is to change your eating habits permanently. If you diet, lose weight, then go back to your old eating habits, your body will gradually regain its lost fat. If you lose weight rapidly, then put it back on again, your body will be flabbier than when you started because some of your muscle mass will have been lost along with the fat.

You become overweight by eating more than you need, and the easiest foods in which to overindulge are fatty and sugary ones. Once you are overweight you only need to eat a very little extra – if any – to service your excess weight.

If you want to lose weight, the first thing to do is to assess what you eat and decide whether you are eating a little too much of *the basic healthy diet* (see pp. 12-13), or whether your diet is over-balanced with fatty and sugary foods. If you became overweight at an earlier stage in your life, but are now eating a healthy diet, then you should cut down your total calorie intake while still eating the same balance of foods. If your diet is faulty, switch to *the basic healthy diet* and see what happens. You may start to lose weight automatically. If not, cut down your calories as explained above.

Exercise
You can influence your weight loss by taking frequent exercise, preferably at least three times a week. This speeds up the rate at which your body burns up calories. When you have reached your target weight, you need to balance the amount of exercise you take with the amount of food you eat.

Little and often
Spread your food intake into five or six meals throughout the day rather than one or two toward the end. Have some breakfast even if you are not used to it. Your body burns up food more quickly earlier in the day.

Pamper yourself
Losing weight is a way of looking after yourself. Take the time to make your meals attractive – you are looking after someone important.

Ten-point plan

This is a safe way of losing weight:

● *Cut down fats, especially animal fat in the form of butter, margarine, dripping, fat on meat, whole milk, cheese, whole milk yoghurt, cream, and any foods made with these ingredients. Use vegetable oils and fats sparingly.*

● *Eat fish or poultry instead of red meat. It is lower in calories.*

● *Cut down added sugar. This means white, brown, and multi-coloured sugar, and any foods made with sugar such as cakes, biscuits, many canned and bottled drinks, and sweetened cereals.*

● *Cut down other refined carbohydrates including non-wholegrain breads; any foods containing refined cereal flour; white rice; and alcohol. Check the ingredients lists of processed foods.*

● *Eat high-fibre foods such as wholegrain bread, cereal and pastas, brown rice, nuts, seeds, pulses (beans and peas), lentils, fruits, and vegetables. Fibre helps fill you up, and levels out blood sugar swings.*

● *Use a good diet or work out your own based on approximately 9 calories per pound (20 calories per kg) of your target body weight per day. Make sure your diet consists of nutritious food (see pp. 12-13).*

● *If you cannot lose weight, you could be sensitive to one or more foods (see* Food sensitivity*). Cereal flour and dairy products are two common "culprits".*

● *If you go off your diet for a day, do not give up. It is the long haul that counts. Be gentle and forgiving with yourself and go back to the diet as soon as you can.*

● *If you overeat as part of your comfort and reward system, think of a substitute. Some successful slimmers find it helps if they do something they really enjoy when they feel a craving to eat.*

● *Aim at weight loss of no more than 1kg (2lb) a week, especially if you have over 3kg (7lb) to lose. Dramatic weight loss in the first week may be caused by fluid loss. Women often find that their weight fluctuates according to their menstrual cycle.*

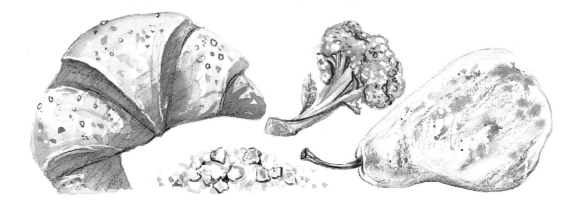

Recommended weights

This chart is for both sexes and is based on up-to-date life insurance statistics that indicate similar recommended weights for men and women of the same height.

Height (without shoes)		Weight (without clothes)				Height (without shoes)		Weight (without clothes)			
		Acceptable		Overweight				Acceptable		Overweight	
m	ft ins	kg	lbs	kg	lbs	m	ft ins	kg	lbs	kg	lbs
1.45	4 9	42-53	92-116	64	141	1.70	5 7	58-73	127-160	88	194
1.48	4 10	42-54	92-119	65	143	1.72	5 8	59-74	130-163	89	196
1.50	4 11	43-55	95-121	66	145	1.74	5 9	60-75	132-165	90	198
1.52	5 0	44-57	97-125	68	149	1.76	5 9	62-77	136-169	92	202
1.54	5 1	44-58	97-127	70	154	1.78	5 10	64-79	141-174	95	209
1.56	5 1	45-58	99-127	70	154	1.80	5 11	65-80	143-176	96	211
1.58	5 2	51-64	112-141	77	169	1.82	6 0	66-82	145-180	98	216
1.60	5 3	52-65	114-143	78	171	1.84	6 0	67-84	147-185	101	222
1.62	5 4	53-66	116-145	79	174	1.86	6 1	69-86	152-189	103	226
1.64	5 5	54-67	119-147	80	176	1.88	6 2	71-88	156-194	106	231
1.66	5 5	55-69	121-152	83	182	1.90	6 3	73-90	160-198	108	237
1.68	5 6	56-71	123-156	85	187	1.92	6 4	75-93	165-205	112	246

How overweight are you?

Three degrees of overweight are shown. First degree does not affect health, but life expectancy is slightly reduced. Second degree may cause shortness of breath, fatigue on exercise, and proneness to *diabetes, high blood pressure, gallbladder* disease, *gout*, lung disorders, osteoarthritis, hernias, and *varicose veins*. Life expectancy can fall, mainly because of heart disease. Operations are more risky. People with third degree overweight have the same problems, but more so.

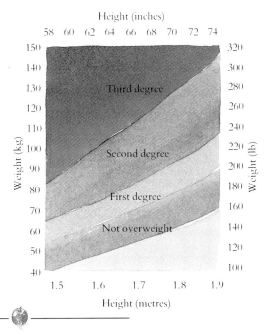

The semi-fast diet

A short time on a semi-fast may help you feel generally better, and it can be a great pick-me-up if you are chronically tired. It is better to start the diet on a day when you do not have to exert yourself physically.

If you have rheumatoid *arthritis* or *high blood pressure*, you may benefit from a regular semi-fast one day a week. This is also a good way to initiate the dietary treatment of *candidiasis*, and some holistic *cancer* specialists recommend an occasional semi-fast. Some conditions, such as migraine, or *diabetes* which is being treated with drugs, might be adversely affected by a semi-fast. Check with your doctor first.

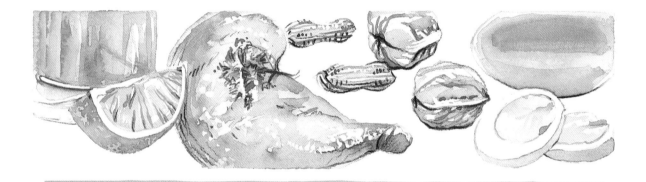

Day 1 *Drink a glass of freshly squeezed or pressed fruit and/or vegetable juice at approximately four-hourly intervals. Quench your thirst with mineral water or herb tea, and make sure you drink at least 1½ litres (3 pints) of fluid during the day. Some suggested juices are apple, orange, grape, pineapple, grapefruit, cranberry, blackcurrant, mango, carrot, beetroot, and celery. A juice extractor is a help for making fresh juice from the harder fruits and vegetables.*

Day 2 *As for Day 1, but add raw and cooked vegetables, and fruit.*

Day 3 *As for Day 2, but add wholegrain cereals, nuts, and seeds.*

Day 4 *As for Day 3, but add fish.*

Day 5 *As for Day 4, but add dairy products and, if you like, meat and eggs. You should now be eating the basic healthy diet.*

The exclusion diet

How to identify "culprit" foods
Food history
Try to link your symptoms with particular foods – did they affect you as a child? Both a craving for and a dislike of a food indicate possible food sensitivity. Record all you consume, and when you experience symptoms, for at least a month. Some symptoms may take up to 4 days to appear – others may appear within minutes. Symptoms usually last less than 24 hours (except eczema, which may last up to 3 weeks).

Individual elimination of suspects
If you suspect a food (or foods), stop eating it. Do not eat it for at least a week and, if there is no change, for up to 3 weeks. If it's a culprit, you will see an improvement between 1 day and 3 weeks. The timing depends on the symptom, the food, and you as an individual.

Positive signs
A quick weight loss of 2.3kg (5lb) or more in the first week, together with the loss or improvement of symptoms, means that you are on the right track. Another positive sign is the worsening of symptoms in the first 3 to 5 days. If neither happens, either the food is not a "culprit" or it is one of several. Now try eliminating the next most likely "culprit".

Challenging
To pinpoint the "culprit", "challenge" with that food. Eat a normal helping between 5 and 12 days after the symptoms have gone. If they reappear, this confirms that the food is the "culprit". Stop eating it and let the reaction pass before challenging with that food again. Ideally, do 3 challenges. Symptoms may be worse than originally. Do not delay a challenge for more than 3 weeks.

IMPORTANT
- *If your symptoms are severe, do not try to pinpoint your "culprit" foods by yourself – consult your doctor.*
- *Do not eliminate a food that is nutritionally important unless you know how to replace it – consult your doctor.*
- *If you have high blood pressure and are on drugs, consult your doctor first.*
- *Check you are eating the basic healthy diet.*
- *There may be cross-sensitivity between foods in the same "family". For a clear result eliminate all members.*

Families of foods

● *Milk and beef family* Beef, suet, beef stock cubes and meat extracts, milk chocolate, dairy foods, casein, whey powder, milk solids, lactalbumen.

● *Wheat family* Wheat grains, flour, or wheat bran, semolina, some breakfast cereals.

● *Potato family* Potatoes, tomatoes, aubergines (eggplants), peppers (cayenne, chillies, paprika, pimento).

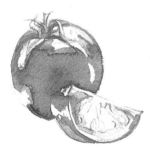

● *Chicken family* Chicken, chicken stock cubes, eggs, lecithin.

● *Caffeine family* Coffee, tea, chocolate, cocoa, cola.

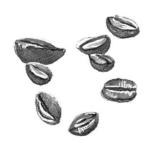

● *Salicylate family* Colourings, benzoates, hydrozybenzoates, gallates, trihydroxybenzoates; apples, apricots, avocados, berries, blackcurrants, cherries, currants, dates, figs, grapes, grapefruit, lemons, marrows, melons, peaches, plums, prunes, oranges, passion fruit, pears with skins, pineapples, raisins, rhubarb, sultanas; asparagus, aubergines (eggplants), broad and green beans, beetroot, broccoli, carrots, courgettes (zucchini), cucumbers, mushrooms, olives, onions, parsnips, peppers, potatoes in their skins, radishes, spinach, sweetcorn, sweet potatoes, tomatoes, turnips, watercress; aniseed, celery seed, cinnamon, cumin, curry, dill, fenugreek, garam masala, mace, mustard, oregano, paprika, rosemary, sage, tarragon, turmeric, thyme; cola, coffee, tea, peppermint tea, most fruit juice, alcohol; almonds, brazil nuts, peanuts, pine nuts, pistachios, sesame seeds, walnuts, water chestnuts; honey, liquorice, peppermints, yeast, wine and cider vinegar.
N.B. People sensitive to salicylates may also be sensitive to tartrazine.

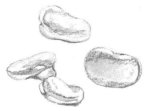

● *Gluten family* Wheat (including "gluten-free" flour, which may contain a little gluten), barley, oats, and rye grains, and flour.

● *Yeast family* Brewer's and baker's yeast, alcohol, bread (except chappatis and matzos), some buns, cheese, yoghurt, buttermilk, soured cream, synthetic cream, yeast extract, stock cubes, beef extract, dried fruits, malt, malted drinks, vinegar, pickled foods, overripe or mouldy foods, grapes, mushrooms, fruit juices (unless freshly squeezed).
N.B. Foods left in warm, moist conditions may be contaminated with yeasts.

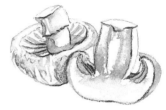

● *Corn family* Corn (maize), sweetcorn, corn oil, blended vegetable oil, glucose syrup, dextrose, baking powder, foods containing cornflour or corn syrup, bottled sauces, baked beans, cornflakes, custard powder, margarine, popcorn, polenta, tortillas.

● *Tartrazine family* Some fruit drinks, carbonated, and fizzy drinks, pickles, bottled sauces, shop cakes, cake mix, packet and canned soups, custard powder, canned custard, instant puddings, sweets, filled chocolates, jelly, ice cream, ice lollies, jam, mustard.

● *Sulphur dioxide family* Salads and fruit salads in restaurants (from "stay-fresh" bisulphate spray), wines, chilled fruit juices, pickled onions, dried fruits, commercial pre-cut chips (french fries).

Modified exclusion diet for adults

The commonest "culprit" foods are eliminated all at once, then added back by challenging (see p. 91). Add back the commonest foods first, one by one, every 3 to 7 days. Do this diet under a doctor's supervision.

	Excluded	Included
Meat	Beef, pork, bacon, preserved meats, sausages, chicken	Lamb, turkey, rabbit, game
Fish	Smoked fish, shellfish	White fish (unless you have eczema)
Vegetables	Potatoes, onions, sweetcorn, soya, tomatoes	Spinach, swede, celery, lettuce, leeks, peas, lentils, beans (except broad and green), brussels sprouts, cabbage. (No beans, lentils, brussels sprouts or cabbage if you have bowel symptoms.)
Fruit	All except (see right)	Bananas, peeled pears, mangoes, pomegranates, paw-paws
Cereals	Wheat, oats, barley, rye, corn	Rice, ground rice, rice flakes, rice flour, rice cakes, rice cereals, sago, tapioca, millet, buckwheat
Cooking oils	Corn, soya, vegetable, nut	Sunflower, safflower, olive, linseed
Dairy products	Cows' milk, butter, margarine, cows' milk yoghurt and cheese, all goat, sheep, and soya milk products	Non-dairy margarines
Beverages	Tea, coffee, "fruit" drinks, orange juice, grapefruit juice, alcohol, tap water	Herbal teas, mineral, distilled, de-ionized or filtered water (use a water filter)
Other	Eggs, chocolate, yeast, herbs, preservatives, additives, spices, sugar, honey	Sea salt

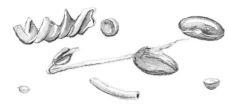

Index

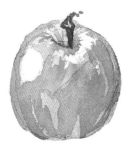

Also published by Gaia Books

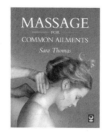

Massage for Common Ailments
Sara Thomas
£8.99
ISBN 1 85675 031 0
Simple massage techniques for effective
and precise treatment of everyday problems,
both physical and mental.

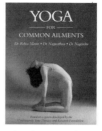

Yoga for Common Ailments
Dr R Monro, Dr Nagarathna and Dr Nagendra
£7.99
ISBN 1 85675 010 8
Simple sequences of yoga postures to
counteract common disorders. Design a
programme for your personal needs.

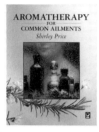

Aromatherapy for Common Ailments
by Shirley Price
ISBN 1 85675 005 1
£7.99
Essential oils cleanse the body, release
physical and mental tension, and balance
the mind. The beautiful photography
and informative text from best-selling
author Shirley Price provide an
invaluable reference on treating a wide
range of ailments.

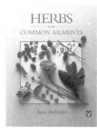

Herbs for Common Ailments
by Anne McIntyre
ISBN 1 85675 055 8
£7.99
The value of herbs has been known since the
dawn of civilisation. Herbs for Common
Ailments responds to today's renewed search
for simple, effective and natural treatments.
It shows how to choose and use herbs for
everyday illnesses.

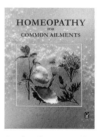

Homeopathy for Common Ailments
by Robin Hayfield
ISBN 1 85675 021 3
£7.99
Homeopathic remedies are safe,
natural forms of treatment.
This book helps you select
remedies for physical and emotional
problems, from coughs and croup to
anxiety, chicken pox, bites and stings and
hayfever. Ideal for children's treatments.

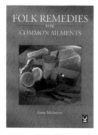

Folk Remedies for Common Ailments
by Anne McIntyre
ISBN 1 85675 086 8
£8.99
Successful and reliable cures for nearly 300
conditions. An invaluable resource for self
help, prevention and first aid from your
kitchen, bathroom or hedgerow.

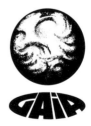

For a catalogue of titles published by Gaia
Books, write or telephone
Gaia Books, 20 High Street, Stroud,
Gloucestershire
GL5 1AS.
Tel 01453 752985 Fax 01453 752987